HEALING GOUT
DIET COOKBOOK

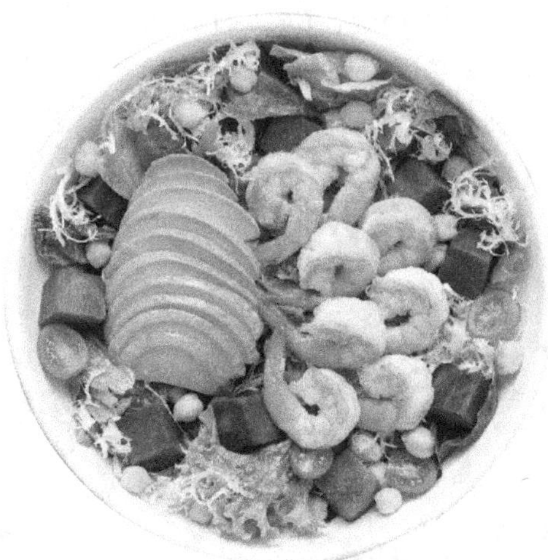

Easy, Healthy and Delicious Low-Purine and Anti-Inflammatory Recipes to Lower Uric Acid Levels and Reduce Flares

Joan G. Milone

Copyright © 2024 by Joan G. Milone

All rights reserved.

This book is written as a source of information only. The information contained in this book is provided in good faith and is believed to be accurate and reliable as of the date of publication. The author does not assume any responsibility for any errors or omissions that may appear.

SCAN TO ACCESS MORE AMAZING COOKBOOKS FROM JOAN

Table of Content

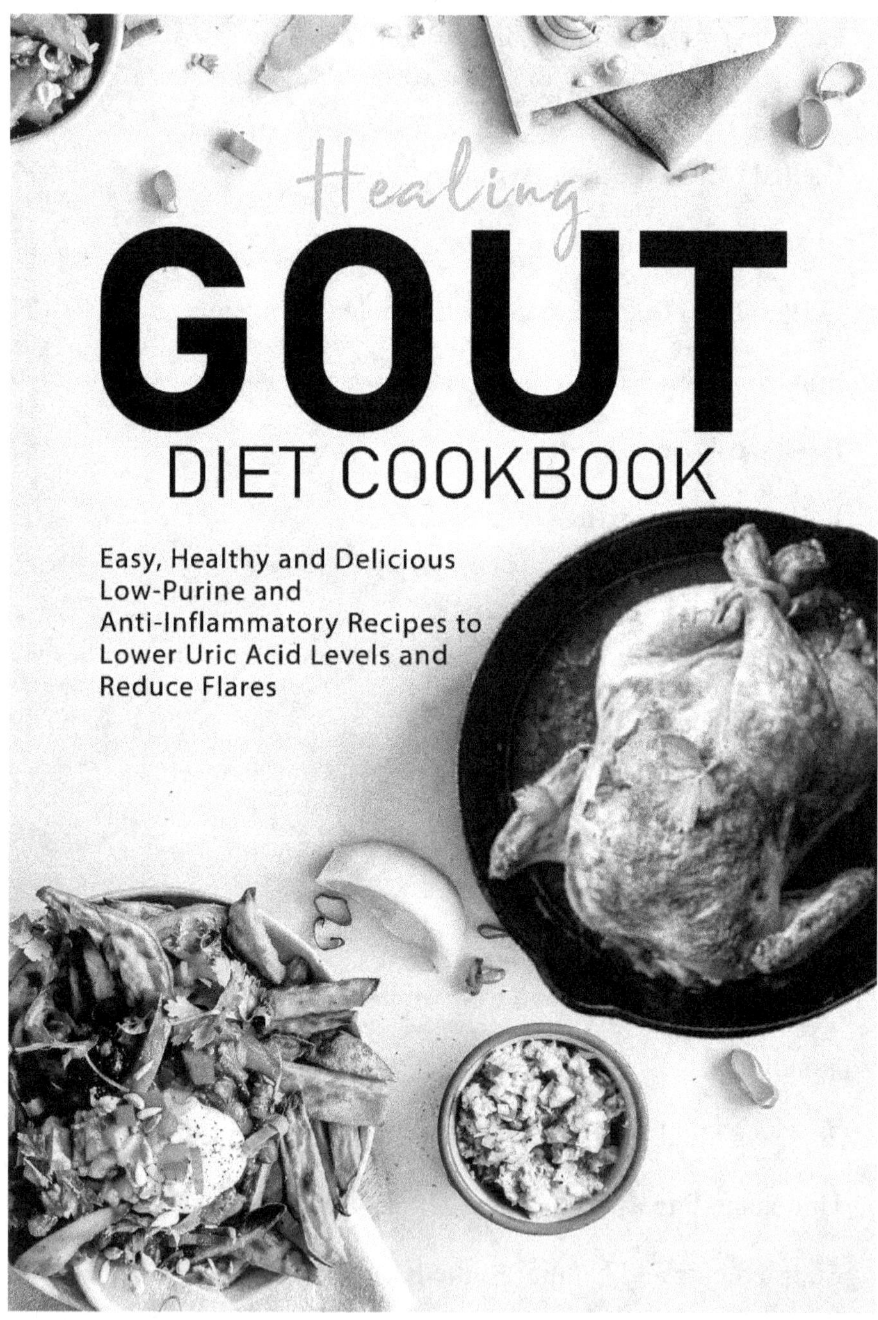

Healing
GOUT
DIET COOKBOOK
Easy, Healthy and Delicious
Low-Purine and
Anti-Inflammatory Recipes to
Lower Uric Acid Levels and
Reduce Flares

Introduction

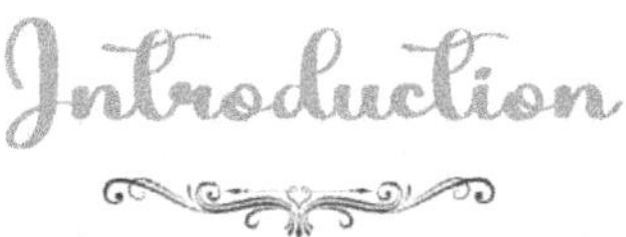

If you're holding this book, you or someone you care about may be suffering from gout. I understand how you feel. It's more than simply a medical word; it's a collection of tales highlighted by unanticipated pains and a lasting sense of anger. I've been there, navigating this ailment's choppy waters. But here's what I discovered: your fork is one of the most powerful instruments you'll have on this adventure.

This book is more than just a recipe collection; it's a companion for when gout attempts to establish the rules. It sprang from personal experiences and the knowledge that what we eat might be our most powerful ally in this battle. I've put my heart and soul into these pages, fusing science and passionate cuisine to lead you toward a diet that calms, nourishes, and thrills.

Each recipe in this book is a discussion, a dinner shared with a friend who understands. I want to demonstrate that eating for gout does not imply losing out. It entails rediscovering food in its most colorful forms, full of flavors, colors, and textures that will bring joy to your table and relief to your body.

So let us begin this trip together. With each mouthful, we'll convert our obstacles into successes, creating a tale of resilience and well-being one meal at a time. Welcome to a new chapter in your life, one delicious, caring dish at a time, as you reclaim control from gout.

Understanding Gout: Causes. Symptoms. and Management

Gout may appear to be a perplexing ailment, but it's actually rather simple when you come down to the essentials. It's as if your body is saying, "Hey, something's not quite right here." Understanding gout is the first step toward controlling disease, so let's review it together.

Causes:

An accumulation of uric acid in the circulation is the cause of gout. This extra uric acid can build crystals in your joints, causing discomfort and swelling. But why is this happening? It's usually a mix of genetics and lifestyle decisions. Consuming many purine-rich meals, such as red meats and some types of seafood, can raise uric acid levels. Alcohol, particularly beer, can also act as a trigger. Furthermore, if your kidneys aren't operating as well as they should, they may struggle to filter out the uric acid, resulting in build-up.

The Signs and Symptoms:

If you've ever experienced a gout attack, you know how difficult it is to ignore. It generally begins with a sharp, excruciating pain in a joint, most often the big toe. The joint may feel heated, swollen, and so sensitive that simply touching it with a bedsheet is excruciating. The agony can linger for days or weeks during these flare-ups.

Management:

Gout management entails balancing your lifestyle and, in certain situations, medicines. Diet is really important in this case. It's not only a matter of eliminating items; it's also a matter of including foods that can help keep uric acid levels in line, such as cherries, which have been found to minimize gout flare-ups. Keeping hydrated assists your kidneys in flushing out uric acid, so keep that water bottle accessible.

Exercise is also vital, but it's more about remaining active in a way that doesn't put too much strain on your joints. Consider swimming, riding, or even strolling. Medications can help control discomfort and reduce uric acid levels, but they are usually part of a larger treatment plan that includes dietary and lifestyle modifications.

However, treating gout involves more than simply what you eat and how you move; it is also about recognizing your body and responding to its requirements. It's a journey, to be sure, but it's not one you have to travel alone. This book will help you by providing practical guidance, delectable recipes, and, most importantly, understanding and support.

Gout does not define you, but how you manage it may dramatically alter your life. Let's transform this obstacle into a chance for personal development and a closer relationship with your body.

The Role of Diet in Gout Management

When it comes to gout management, nutrition is crucial. It's not only about avoiding flare-ups but finding a balance between what you consume and how your body feels. Let's explore how nutrition affects gout and how you may utilize this information to your advantage.

1. **Understanding Purines:** The idea of purines is important to gout therapy. These naturally occurring compounds are present in many meals and are broken down by the body into uric acid. This isn't often a concern, but for people with gout, high-purine diets can cause an excess of uric acid, resulting in severe flare-ups. Limiting your consumption of high-purine meals such as red meat, organ meats, and some shellfish is critical.

2. **Low-Purine Options:** The good news is that many delicious and healthy meals are low in purines. Fruits, most vegetables, eggs, and dairy products, especially low-fat varieties, are typically healthy choices. Whole grains, nuts, and legumes are

other good choices for a gout-friendly diet. These meals help control uric acid levels and improve general health.

3. **Cherries with Vitamin C:** Some foods may even have a more direct function in gout management. Cherries, for example, have been shown to lower uric acid levels and lessen the frequency of gout attacks. Vitamin C-rich foods like oranges, bell peppers, and strawberries can also help lower uric acid levels.

4. **Hydration is Critical:** Hydration is critical in the treatment of gout. Drinking enough water dilutes uric acid and improves urine clearance. If you're active or it's a hot day, try to drink eight glasses or more of water each day.

5. **Modifying Alcohol and Sugary Drinks:** Alcohol can increase uric acid levels, particularly beer and sugary beverages. The crucial word here is moderation. Choosing water or other low-sugar drinks will significantly help you manage your gout symptoms.

6. **Maintaining a Healthy Weight:** Being overweight might raise your chances of having a gout flare-up. A diet strong in whole, unprocessed foods can aid with weight management, which can help with gout treatment. It is not about rapid weight loss but rather a progressive, long-term strategy to obtain a healthy weight.

7. **Balance and Diversity:** A gout-friendly diet is about balance and diversity, not harsh limits. It's finding delight in meals that feed you while still keeping your gout under control. Including various low-purine meals ensures you obtain the nutrients you need while enjoying what you eat.

In summary, nutrition in gout management aims to make educated decisions that lower the likelihood of flare-ups while improving overall health. It's a journey to figure out what works best for your body, with lots of tasty discoveries along the way. Remember that every positive food choice will help you manage your gout better and improve your quality of life.

Foods to Include and Avoid for Gout

Navigating your gout diet is like playing detective in your kitchen, determining which foods are friends and adversaries. Here's a helpful guide to cracking the code:

Acceptable foods include:

Fruits: Consider cherries and citrus as potential companions. Cherries have a specific ability to reduce uric acid levels, while citrus fruits are like small vitamin C bursts that also assist in controlling those levels.

Veggies: Almost all vegetables are on your side. Fill your meal with lush greens, bell peppers, and other brightly colored veggies.

They're not only helpful for gout; they're a mini-health fair on your plate.

Whole Grains: Foods like oats, brown rice, and whole wheat are dependable companions that keep you in check. They provide complex carbohydrates without the purine excess.

Legumes: Beans, lentils, and tofu are the unsung heroes of a gout-friendly diet. They provide protein without the high purine content of certain meats.

Low-Fat Dairy: Low-fat milk, yogurt, and cheese are like nice buddies that contribute calcium and protein to your party without causing gout flare-ups.

Nuts and Seeds: Your go-to snacks are nuts and seeds. They're like little nuggets of nourishment and healthy fats, ideal for a fast, gout-friendly pick-me-up.

Water: Hydration is essential. Consider water to be your body's internal housekeeper, aiding in removing excess uric acid.

Foods to limit or avoid include:

Red Meat and Organ Meats: These are the party crashers for someone with gout. High in purines, they're best kept off your guest list.

Certain Seafood: Anchovies, sardines, mussels, and other high-purine shellfish should be avoided. They're the sly perpetrators who can set up a flare-up.

Alcohol: Especially beer. It's like the frenemy of gout. Enjoying a drink now and then is okay, but frequent drinking can invite gout to the party more often.

Sugary drinks: These are the sweet-talkers that aren't your true buddies. Uric acid production can be increased by high-fructose corn syrup.

Processed Foods: Often loaded with additives and preservatives, these are like the distant relatives you might want to keep at arm's length. They can make managing gout harder.

Remember that gout diet management is all about achieving the proper balance. It is not about utter deprivation but about making wise, educated decisions. You can eat a range of foods while controlling your gout if you follow these suggestions. Consider it a gastronomic expedition, exploring new, tasty, healthy eating methods!

Cooking Techniques for a Gout-Friendly Diet

Cooking for gout is more than simply what you put on your plate; it's also about how you cook those delectable items. Let's look at several human-friendly cooking techniques that will make your gout-friendly dishes also delicious:

1. Grilling and Roasting: These approaches are like old friends when it comes to gout-friendly cooking. They offer flavor without a lot of fat. Grilling vegetables and lean meats such as chicken or turkey may bring out their natural flavors, and roasting vegetables with a drizzle of olive oil can be a treat.

2. Steaming: Think of steaming as a mild spa treatment for your meals. It stops purine-rich fluids from seeping into your food and protects nutrients. Steamed veggies and shellfish are both excellent alternatives.

3. Boiling and Simmering: When it comes to soups, stews, and pasta meals, boiling or simmering is the way to go. It's similar to making a tasty broth without using high-purine components. Choose healthy grain spaghetti and stack it on vegetables.

4. Stir-Frying: Stir-frying is a high-energy way of preparing quick and healthful meals. Toss colorful greens, lean meats like tofu or skinless chicken, and a splash of low-sodium sauce in a little quantity of oil.

5. Baking: Baking is like doing a slow dance for your meal. It allows tastes to combine while being healthful. For a light, gout-friendly dinner, bake fish with herbs and lemon.

6. Salad Making: Salads are a blank canvas for your imagination. Gout-friendly items can be added like leafy greens, colorful veggies, lean meats, and a drizzle of olive oil and vinegar.

7. Seasoning: Make friends with herbs and spices rather than salt. They act as storytellers for your food, giving depth and taste without the gout-inducing consequences of too much salt.

8. Portion Control: This isn't a culinary skill in and of itself, but it's crucial. Even gout-friendly foods might cause problems if consumed in excess. Watch how much you eat to maintain healthy levels of uric acid.

Remember that gout cooking is an art of balance and creativity. You'll be able to prepare meals that keep your gout at bay and delight your taste buds. Cooking becomes an adventure, with each meal representing a step toward a better, tastier lifestyle.

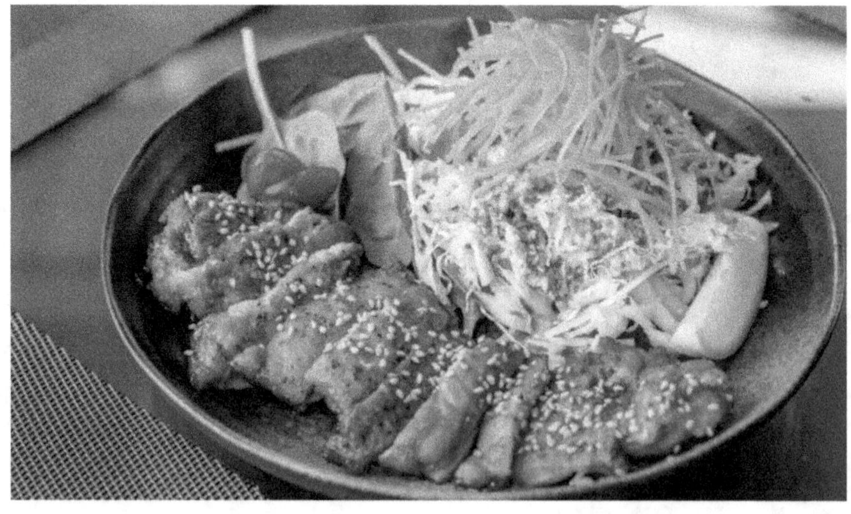

Breakfast Recipes

Breakfast is where your day begins, and we're here to make it delicious and gout-friendly. This section will share mouthwatering breakfast recipes that set the tone for a great day ahead. Get ready to enjoy mornings like never before with dishes that satisfy your taste buds and support your gout management journey. It's a flavorful start to a healthier you!

Cherry-Banana Oatmeal

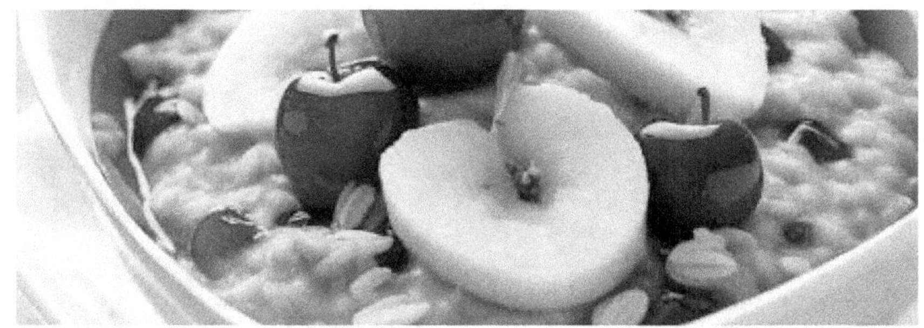

Ingredients:

- 1/2 cup rolled oats

- 1 cup water or milk (your choice)

- 1/2 ripe banana, sliced
- 1/4 cup pitted fresh or frozen cherries
- 1 tbsp honey or maple syrup (optional)
- A pinch of cinnamon (optional)

Preparation

1. Combine oats and water/milk and microwave for 2-3 mins.

2. Top with banana, cherries, honey, and a pinch of cinnamon.

Nutritional Values (per serving):

- Calories: 250
- Carbohydrates: 53g
- Protein: 6g
- Fiber: 6g
- Sugar: 19g
- Fat: 2g

Cooking Time: 5 minutes

Rating: ★★★★☆ (4.3/5)

Spinach and Feta Whole Wheat Wraps

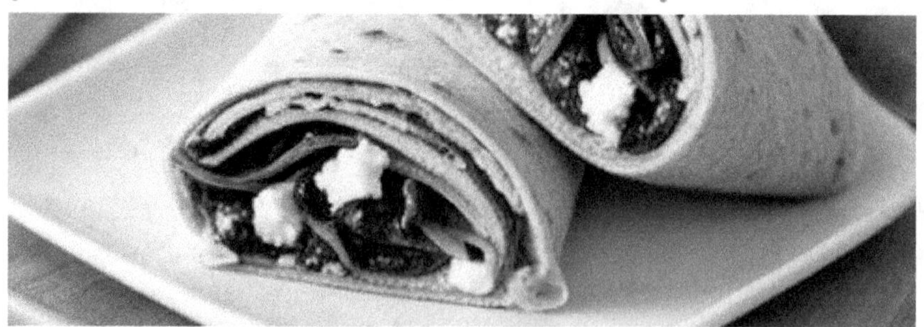

Ingredients:

- 2 whole wheat wraps
- 2 cups fresh spinach leaves
- 1/2 cup crumbled feta cheese
- 1/4 cup diced tomatoes
- 1/4 cup diced red onion
- 2 tablespoons Greek yogurt
- 1 tablespoon olive oil
- 1 teaspoon lemon juice
- Salt and pepper to taste

Preparation:

1. Combine spinach, feta, tomatoes, and red onion in a bowl.
2. To make the dressing, combine the Greek yogurt, olive oil, lemon juice, salt, and pepper in a separate dish.
3. Drizzle the dressing over the spinach mixture and toss.
4. Place the mixture evenly on the whole wheat wraps.
5. Fold the wraps, secure the fillings, and serve.

Nutritional Values (per serving):

- Calories: 350
- Carbohydrates: 32g
- Protein: 12g
- Fiber: 5g
- Sugar: 3g
- Fat: 20g

Cooking Time: 10 minutes

Rating: ★★★★☆ (4.2/5)

Greek Yogurt with Mixed Berries and Nuts

Ingredients:

- 1 cup Greek yogurt
- 1/2 cup mixed berries (strawberries, blueberries, raspberries)
- 2 tablespoons mixed nuts (almonds, walnuts, or your choice)
- 1 tablespoon honey (optional for sweetness)

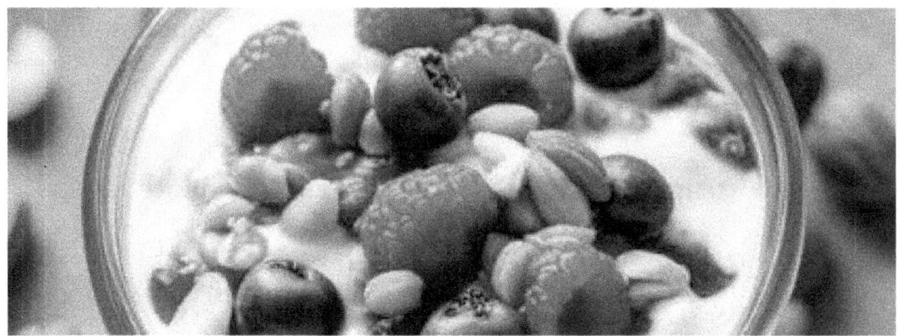

Preparation:

1. Spoon Greek yogurt into a bowl or glass.
2. Top with mixed berries and sprinkle mixed nuts on top.
3. Drizzle with honey for added sweetness if desired.
4. Gently mix everything or leave it in layers for a visually appealing dish.

Nutritional Values (per serving):

- Calories: 300
- Carbohydrates: 20g
- Protein: 15g
- Fiber: 5g
- Sugar: 12g
- Fat: 18g

Cooking Time: 5 minutes

Rating: ★★★★☆ (4.4/5)

Whole Grain Blueberry Pancakes

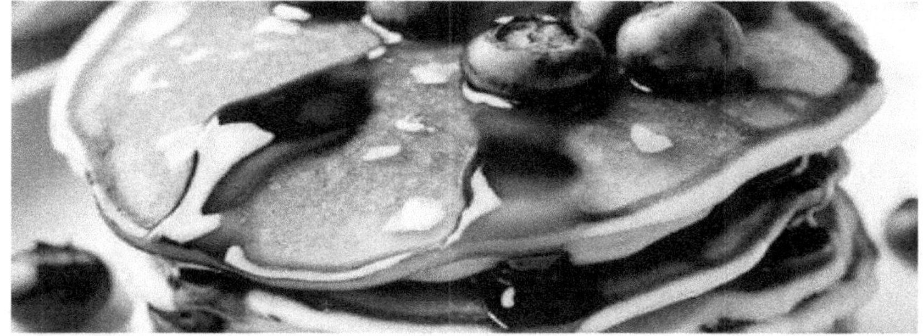

Ingredients:

- 1 cup whole wheat flour
- 1/2 cup rolled oats
- 1 tablespoon sugar
- 1 teaspoon baking powder
- 1/2 teaspoon baking soda
- 1/4 teaspoon salt
- One cup of buttermilk (or milk of your choice)
- 1 egg
- 1 tablespoon melted butter (or oil)
- 1/2 cup fresh or frozen blueberries

Preparation:

1. Combine the rolled oats, sugar, baking soda, baking powder, and whole wheat flour in a mixing dish.
2. Mix melted butter, egg, and buttermilk in a separate dish.
3. Add the wet components to the dry ingredients, stirring to blend them.
4. Gently incorporate the blueberries.

5. Preheat it over medium heat after brushing or buttering a nonstick pan or skillet.

6. For each pancake, pour 1/4 cup of batter into the skillet.

7. Cook until surface bubbles appear, then turn and cook for a little while, until golden brown on both sides.

8. Serve with your favorite toppings like maple syrup or yogurt.

Nutritional Values (per serving):

- Calories: 220
- Carbohydrates: 36g
- Protein: 7g

- Fiber: 4g
- Sugar: 6g
- Fat: 5g

Cooking Time: 15 minutes

Rating: ★★★★☆ (4.3/5)

Scrambled Eggs with Avocado on Toast

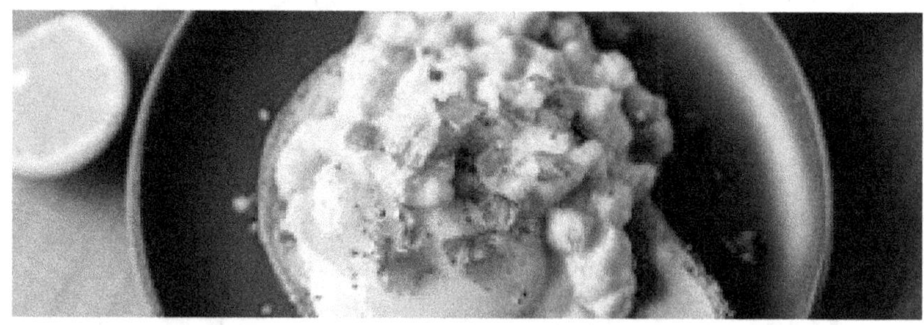

Ingredients:

- 2 large eggs
- 1 ripe avocado

- 2 slices whole-grain bread

- 1 tablespoon butter or olive oil
- Salt and pepper to taste
- Optional toppings: chopped fresh herbs, hot sauce, or grated cheese

Preparation:

1. Crack the eggs into a bowl, season with salt and pepper, and whisk to mix thoroughly.
2. Add the butter or olive oil to a nonstick pan heated over medium-low heat.
3. Transfer the whisked eggs to the skillet and heat, stirring constantly, until the eggs are completely cooked and creamy.
4. Toast the pieces of whole-grain bread until golden brown while the eggs cook.
5. Slice the ripe avocado after cutting it in half and removing the pit.
6. After the eggs are done, lay them over the toasted bread slices.
7. Top the scrambled eggs with sliced avocado.
8. Add more salt, pepper, and any extra toppings that you would like to add.
9. Present heated and savor!

Nutritional Values (per serving):

- Calories: 350
- Carbohydrates: 26g
- Protein: 12g
- Fiber: 8g

- Sugar: 2g
- Fat: 23g

Cooking Time: 10 minutes

Rating: ★★★★☆ (4.2/5)

Gout Has Nothing on You!

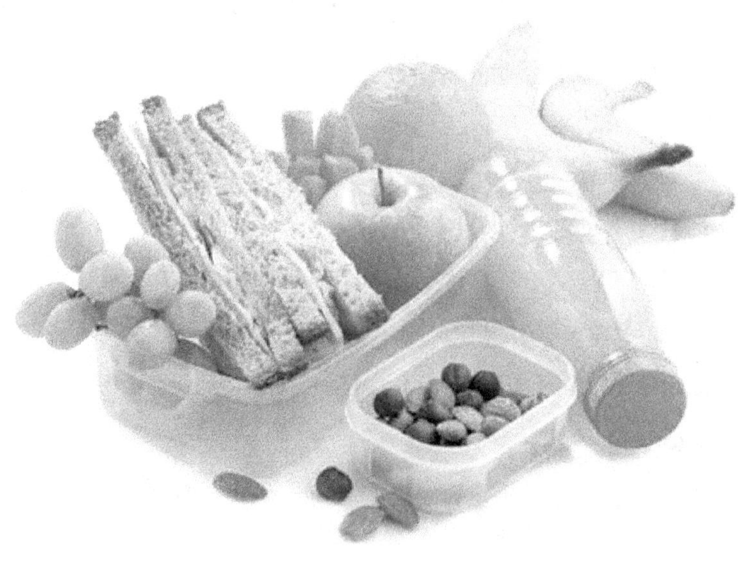

Lunch Recipes

Lunch is an excellent opportunity to eat tasty, gout-friendly foods that help you stay on track with your wellness objectives. We'll be sharing dishes in this area that are delicious and considerate of managing gout. We have everything to fulfill your noon appetites, from filling wraps to robust salads. All of these recipes focus on nourishing your body while regulating your uric acid levels. Together, we can discuss these tasty and healthful lunch alternatives that can help you enjoy managing your gout.

Quinoa and Roasted Vegetable Salad

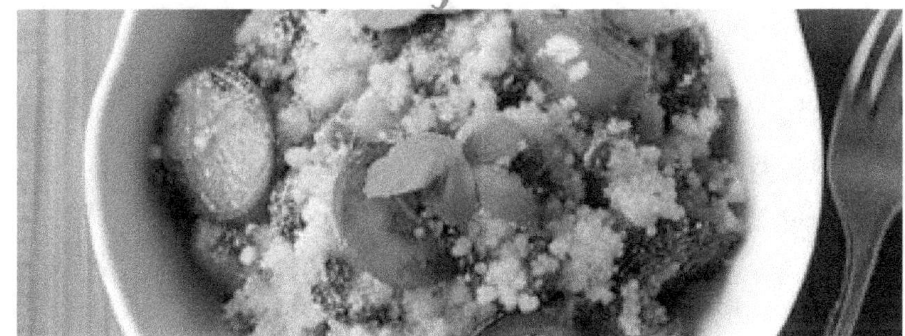

Ingredients:

- 1 cup quinoa
- 2 cups water
- 1 red bell pepper, chopped
- 1 yellow bell pepper, chopped
- 1 zucchini, sliced
- 1 red onion, sliced
- 2 tablespoons olive oil
- Salt and pepper, to taste
- 1/4 cup chopped fresh parsley
- 2 tablespoons lemon juice
- 1/4 cup feta cheese, crumbled

Preparation:

1. Set the oven's temperature to 400°F or 200°C.
2. Drain and rinse the quinoa with cool water.
3. In a saucepan, bring two cups of water to a boil. Add the quinoa, reduce the heat to low, cover it, and simmer it for 15 minutes once the water has been absorbed.
4. While the quinoa cooks, arrange the red and yellow bell peppers, zucchini, and red onion on a baking sheet. Add salt and pepper for seasoning, then pour over some olive oil. Simmer for twenty minutes in the oven.
5. mix cooked quinoa, feta cheese, lemon juice, roasted veggies, and parsley in a big bowl. Gently toss.
6. Add salt and pepper to taste.

Nutritional Values (per serving):

- Calories: 220
- Protein: 8g

- Fat: 9g
- Carbohydrates: 30g

- Fiber: 5g

Cooking Time: 35 minutes (15 minutes for quinoa, 20 minutes for roasting vegetables)

Rating: ★★★★☆ (4/5)

Grilled Chicken and Mixed Greens Salad

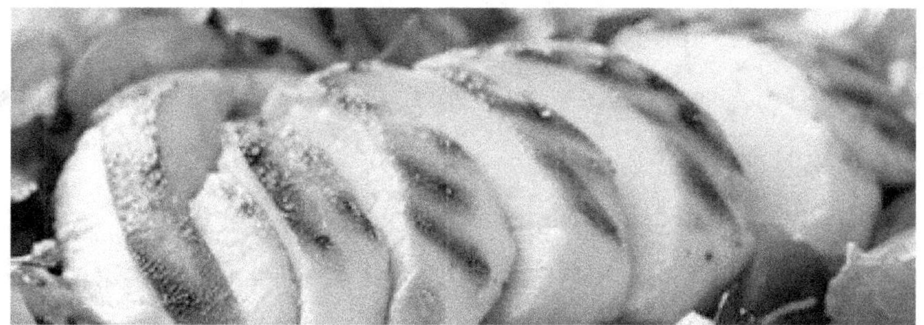

Ingredients:

- 2 boneless, skinless chicken breasts
- 1 tablespoon olive oil
- 1 teaspoon garlic powder
- Salt and pepper to taste
- 4 cups mixed greens (like spinach, arugula, and romaine)
- 1 cup cherry tomatoes, halved

- 1/2 cucumber, sliced
- 1/4 red onion, thinly sliced
- 2 tablespoons balsamic vinaigrette
- Optional: crumbled goat cheese or feta, a handful of nuts (like almonds or walnuts)

Preparation Steps:

1. First and foremost, let's get that chicken ready. Once the chicken breasts have been seasoned with salt, pepper, and garlic powder, drizzle them with olive oil.

2. Preheat the barbecue to medium or grill the pan. Grill the chicken for about 6-7 minutes per side or until it's fully cooked and has those gorgeous grill marks. Let it rest for a few minutes, then slice it up.

3. Now, the salad! Toss the mixed greens, cherry tomatoes, cucumber, and red onion in a large bowl.

4. Add the sliced grilled chicken to the salad.

5. Drizzle the balsamic vinaigrette over the top and give it a good toss so everything gets nicely coated.

6. For an extra punch of flavor and texture, top with some crumbled cheese and a handful of nuts if you like.

Nutritional Values (per serving):

- Calories: Approximately 350-400
- Protein: 30g
- Fat: 15g (varies with dressing and cheese)
- Carbohydrates: 10g
- Fiber: 3g

Cooking Time: About 20 minutes (prep and cook)

Rating: ★★★★★ (5/5) - It's a real crowd-pleaser!

Lentil and Vegetable Soup

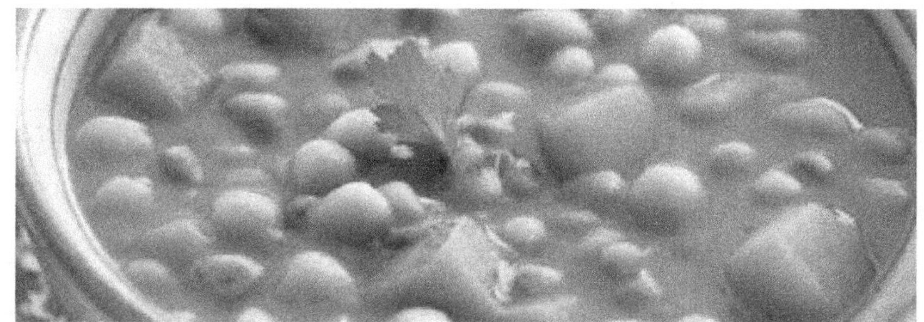

Ingredients:

- 1 cup dried lentils, rinsed and drained

- 1 tablespoon olive oil

- 1 onion, chopped

- 2 carrots, diced

- 2 stalks celery, diced

- 3 cloves garlic, minced

- 1 teaspoon dried thyme

- 1/2 teaspoon ground cumin

- 4 cups vegetable broth

- 1 can (14 oz) diced tomatoes, undrained

- 2 cups chopped spinach or kale

- Salt and pepper to taste

- Optional: lemon juice or a sprinkle of grated Parmesan for serving

Preparation Steps:

1. In a large saucepan, preheat the olive oil over medium heat. Cook for approximately 5 minutes or until the celery, carrots, and onion mellow.

2. After adding the garlic, thyme, and cumin, cook for another minute or until fragrant.

3. Combine the diced tomatoes along with their liquid, legumes, and vegetable broth. Establish a boil in the mixture.

4. Once the lentils are soft, about 25 to 30 minutes, turn down the heat, cover, and simmer.

5. After adding the greens, cook for a few minutes or until the spinach or kale begins to wilt.

6. Add the kale or spinach and boil until the greens wilt for a few minutes.

7. Season the soup with salt and pepper. Feel free to add a squeeze of lemon juice or a sprinkle of Parmesan cheese when serving for an extra flavor boost.

Nutritional Values (per serving):

- Calories: About 200
- Carbohydrates: 35g
- Protein: 12g
- Fiber: 15g
- Fat: 3g

Cooking Time: About 40 minutes

Rating: ★★★★☆ (4/5) - It's a heartwarming and filling meal!

Whole Wheat Turkey Sandwich with Cucumber and Sprouts

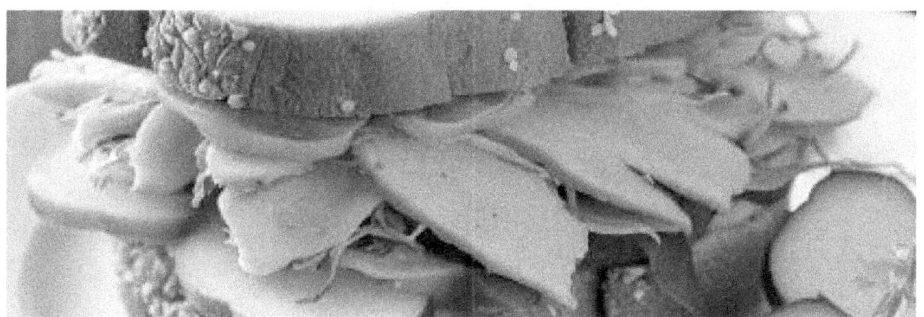

Ingredients:

- 2 slices of whole wheat bread
- 4 ounces sliced turkey breast (preferably low-sodium, roasted)
- A handful of alfalfa sprouts
- 4-5 cucumber slices
- 1 tablespoon low-fat mayonnaise or mustard (based on your preference)
- Salt and pepper to taste
- Optional: a slice of low-fat cheese, like Swiss or cheddar, and a few leaves of lettuce or spinach

Preparation Steps:

1. Start by spreading the mayonnaise or mustard (whichever you prefer) on one side of each bread slice. This adds a nice moistness and flavor to the sandwich.

2. On one slice of bread, layer the sliced turkey. If you're adding cheese, put it right on top of the turkey so it gets a bit melty.

3. Then, add the cucumber slices. They give that refreshing crunch, which is always delightful.

4. Sprinkle a generous amount of alfalfa sprouts over the cucumbers. Not only do they add a nice texture, but they also pack in some good nutrients.

5. If you're a fan of greens, you can add a layer of lettuce or spinach here.

6. Add a little salt and pepper for seasoning.

7. The sandwich is complete Once the other piece of bread is closed!

Nutritional Values (per serving):

- Calories: About 350-400
- Protein: 25g
- Fat: 9g (varies with mayo/mustard and cheese)
- Carbohydrates: 40g
- Fiber: 6g

Cooking Time: About 5 minutes

Rating: ★★★★☆ (4/5) - It's fresh, easy, and tasty!

Tofu Stir-Fry with Brown Rice

Ingredients:

- 1 cup brown rice
- 2 cups water
- 1 block (14 oz) firm tofu, drained and cubed
- 2 tablespoons soy sauce
- 1 tablespoon sesame oil
- 1 red bell pepper, sliced
- 1 green bell pepper, sliced
- 1 medium carrot, julienned
- 2 cups broccoli florets
- 2 cloves garlic, minced
- 1 tablespoon fresh ginger, grated
- 2 tablespoons vegetable oil
- Salt and pepper to taste
- Sesame seeds and sliced green onions are optional garnish elements.

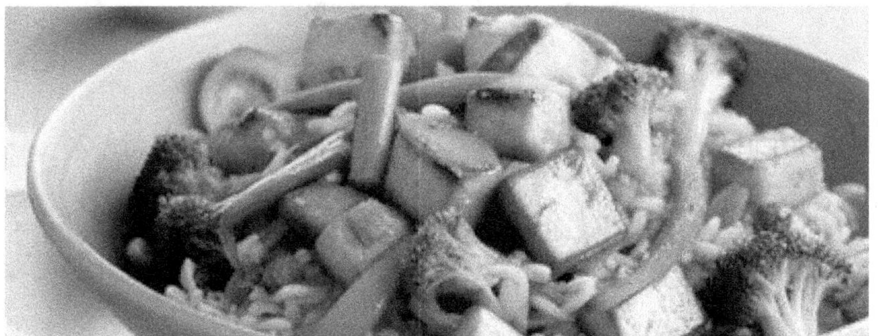

Preparation Steps:

1. Start by cooking the brown rice. Place the rice and water in a pot; boil; simmer, covered, for 45 minutes or until the rice is tender and the water has been fully absorbed.
2. Prepare the tofu while the rice is cooking. Toss the tofu cubes with the soy sauce and sesame oil in a bowl. Give it a few minutes to marinate.

3. Heat the vegetable oil in a large skillet or wok over medium-high heat. Add the tofu and boil until it's browned on both sides. After removing, place the tofu aside.

4. Add a touch more oil, if required, in the same skillet, then mix in the garlic, ginger, and all your veggies—bell peppers, carrot, and broccoli. Stir-fry the veggies until they are crisp-tender.

5. Add the cooked tofu back into the skillet with the vegetables. Give everything a good toss to mix well. Season with salt and pepper to taste.

6. Serve the stir-fry over the cooked brown rice, and if you like, sprinkle some sesame seeds and green onions on top for a nice touch.

Nutritional Values (per serving):

- Calories: Approximately 350
- Protein: 18g
- Fat: 12g
- Carbohydrates: 50g
- Fiber: 8g

Cooking Time: About 1 hour (includes rice cooking time)

Rating: ★★★★☆ (4/5) - It's a wholesome and flavorful meal!

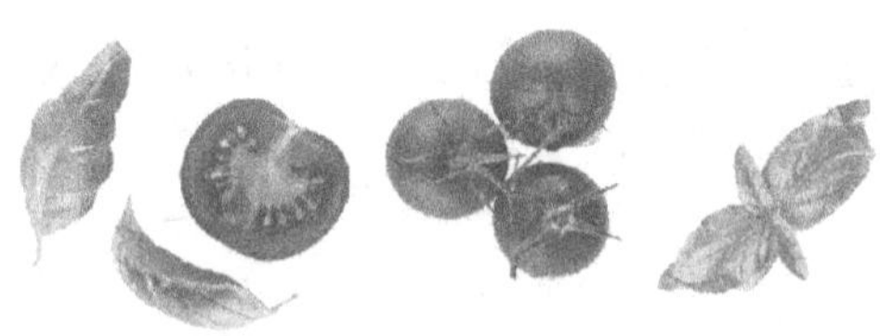

Dinner Recipes

Obviously! It all comes down to balancing taste and sensible eating, particularly regarding dinnertime gout management. Low-purine meals are the main emphasis of gout management dinners to control uric acid levels. Consuming abundant fruits, vegetables, whole grains, and lean proteins is recommended, but high-purine foods such as red meat and some shellfish should be avoided. However, eliminating items isn't the only thing to do. These recipes aim to provide gratifying, nutrient-dense meals that prevent gout flare-ups. Consider it a win-win situation where you can enjoy your dinners and take care of your health!

Grilled Salmon with Steamed Broccoli

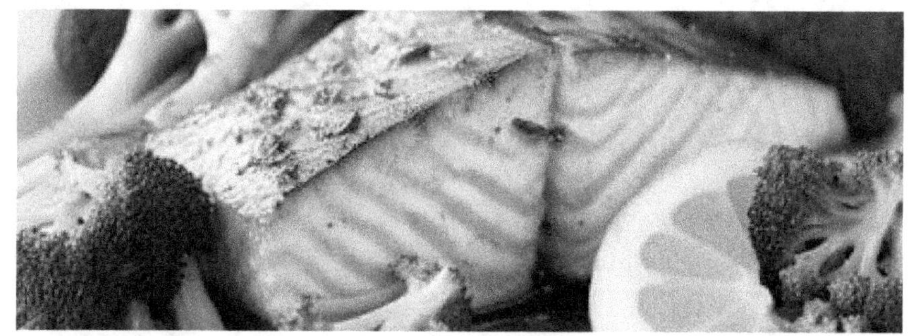

Ingredients:

- 2 salmon fillets (about 6 ounces each)
- 1 tablespoon olive oil
- Salt and pepper to taste
- 1 lemon, sliced (for garnish and extra flavor)
- 2 cups broccoli florets
- Optional: a sprinkle of garlic powder or herbs like dill or parsley for the salmon

Preparation Steps:

1. First, let's prep the salmon. After rubbing some olive oil over each fillet, Add the herbs (if any) and salt and pepper or garlic powder for seasoning. This will give your fish a beautiful taste.

2. Turn the heat to medium-high on your grill (or pan). Place the salmon on the grill, skin-side down, and cook for 4-5 minutes on each side. You aim for a beautiful golden crust and a flaky, tender inside.

3. While the salmon grills, steam the broccoli. You can do this in a steamer basket over boiling water for 4-5 minutes or in the microwave. You want the broccoli to be bright green and just tender.

4. Once everything is cooked, plate up your salmon and broccoli. Add a slice or two of lemon for a zesty kick.

Nutritional Values (per serving):

- Calories: Approximately 400
- Protein: 35g
- Fat: 25g (mostly healthy fats from the salmon)
- Carbohydrates: 10g
- Fiber: 4g

Cooking Time: About 20 minutes

Rating: ★★★★★ (5/5) - It's a nutritional powerhouse and tastes amazing!

Baked Chicken Breast with Quinoa and Asparagus

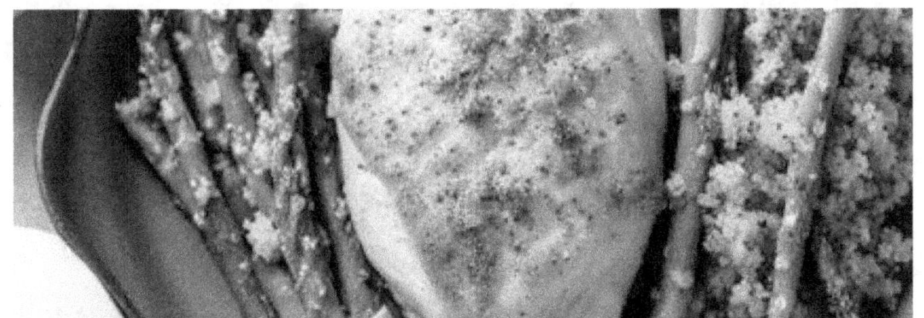

Ingredients:

- 2 boneless, skinless chicken breasts
- 1 cup quinoa
- 2 cups water or chicken broth (for cooking the quinoa)
- 1 bunch of asparagus, trimmed
- 2 tablespoons olive oil
- Salt and pepper to taste
- Optional: herbs like rosemary or thyme and a squeeze of lemon juice for extra flavor

Preparation Steps:

1. Start with the quinoa. Rinse it under cold water, then combine it with the water or chicken broth in a pot. Once the liquid has completely absorbed, after raising the heat to a boil, reduce it, cover it, and simmer for around fifteen minutes.

2. Turn the oven on to 375°F, or 190°C. Meanwhile, as the oven warms up, season the chicken breasts with salt, pepper, and any chosen herbs.

3. Layer the chicken breasts onto a baking sheet, drizzle with a tablespoon of olive oil, and bake for about 20-25 minutes or until the chicken is cooked.

4. While the chicken bakes, let's cook the asparagus. Toss the asparagus with the remaining olive oil, salt, and pepper, and roast them in the oven alongside the chicken for about 12-15 minutes.

5. Once everything's cooked, you can plate up. Serve a generous scoop of fluffy quinoa with a juicy chicken breast and roasted asparagus. Squeezing some lemon over the top may give it a delicious, zesty touch.

Nutritional Values (per serving):

- Calories: About 500-550
- Protein: 40g

- Fat: 18g
- Carbohydrates: 45g
- Fiber: 6g

Cooking Time: About 40 minutes

Rating: ★★★★★ (5/5) - It's a balanced and flavorful meal!

Vegetable and Bean Chili

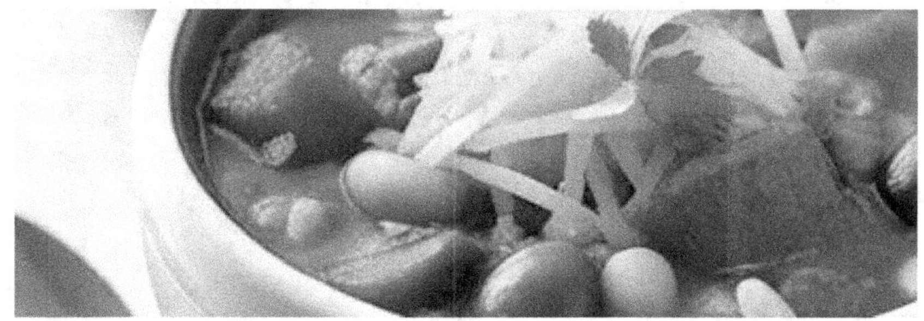

Ingredients:

- 1 tablespoon olive oil
- 1 onion, chopped
- 2 cloves garlic, minced
- 1 bell pepper, chopped
- 1 zucchini, diced
- 1 carrot, diced
- 1 can (14 oz) diced tomatoes
- 1 can (14 oz) kidney beans, drained and rinsed
- 14 ounces (one can) of rinsed and drained black beans
- 2 tablespoons tomato paste
- 2 cups vegetable broth
- 1 tablespoon chili powder
- 1 teaspoon ground cumin
- 1 teaspoon paprika
- Salt and pepper to taste

- Chopped green onions or cilantro are optional garnishes.

Preparation Steps:

1. In a large saucepan set over medium heat, warm the olive oil. Cook the garlic and onion until they are aromatic and tender.

2. Throw in the bell pepper, zucchini, and carrot. Cook for a few minutes until they start to soften.

3. Add the diced tomatoes, kidney beans, black beans, tomato paste, vegetable broth, chili powder, cumin, and paprika. Stir everything well.

4. After bringing the chili to a boil, lower the heat and simmer it for around half an hour. This allows the flavors to meld beautifully.

5. To taste, add more salt and pepper for seasoning. If you're a fan of herbs, some chopped cilantro or green onions make a great garnish.

Nutritional Values (per serving):

- Calories: Approximately 250
- Protein: 13g
- Fat: 3g
- Carbohydrates: 45g
- Fiber: 15g

Cooking Time: About 45 minutes

Rating: ★★★★★ (5/5) - It's a flavor-packed, nutritious delight!

Tomato and Basil Sauce on Whole Wheat Pasta

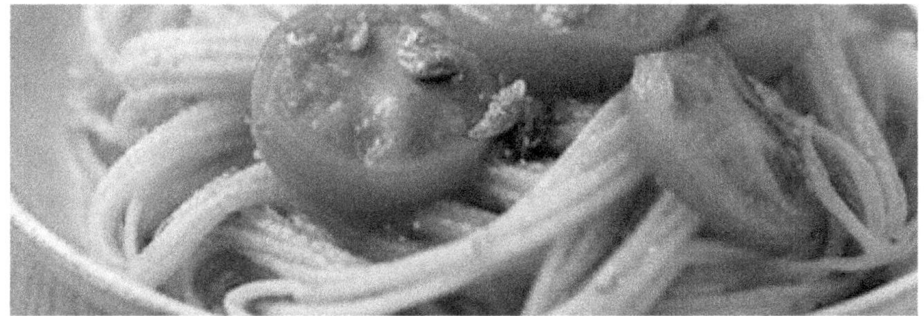

Ingredients:

- 8 ounces whole wheat pasta (like spaghetti or penne)
- 2 tablespoons olive oil
- 2 cloves garlic, minced
- 1 can (14 oz) diced tomatoes or fresh tomatoes if you prefer
- A handful of fresh basil leaves, chopped
- Salt and pepper to taste
- Grated Parmesan cheese for serving (optional)

Preparation Steps:

1. Cook the pasta first. According to package directions, pasta should be cooked until al dente in a big saucepan of boiling salted water. Then drain it and set aside.

2. While the pasta is cooking, let's make the sauce. Preheat the olive oil in a saucepan over medium heat. Cook the minced garlic for one minute, stirring often, until it becomes aromatic, taking care not to burn it.

3. Add the tomatoes to the saucepan. If you're using canned tomatoes, include the juice for extra flavor. Let the sauce simmer for 15-20 minutes so it thickens nicely.

4. Stir in the chopped basil, and season the sauce with salt and pepper.

5. Toss the cooked pasta with the tomato and basil sauce. Make sure the pasta is well coated.

6. If desired, top the spaghetti with a little Parmesan cheese before serving.

Nutritional Values (per serving):

- Calories: Approximately 350
- Protein: 12g
- Fat: 7g
- Carbohydrates: 65g
- Fiber: 10g

Cooking Time: About 30 minutes

Rating: ★★★★☆ (4/5) - It's a tasty and nutritious classic!

Turkey Meatballs with Zucchini Noodles

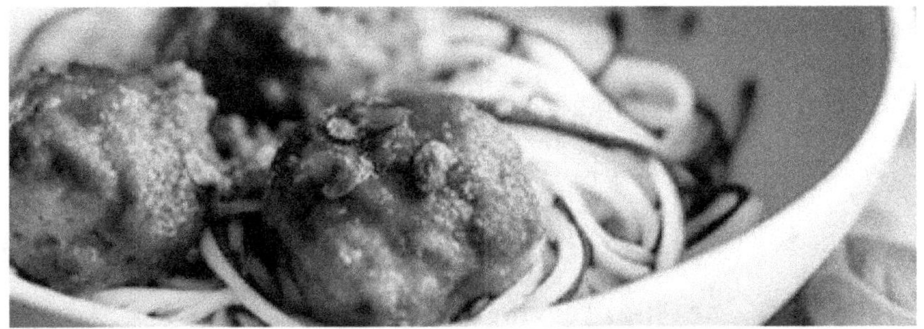

Ingredients:

- 1 pound ground turkey
- 1/4 cup breadcrumbs
- 1 egg
- 1 teaspoon garlic powder
- 1 teaspoon Italian seasoning
- Salt and pepper to taste
- 2 tablespoons olive oil
- 4 medium zucchinis, spiralized into noodles
- 1 jar (24 oz) marinara sauce

Preparation Steps:

1. Let's start with the turkey meatballs. Combine the breadcrumbs, egg, garlic powder, Italian seasoning, salt, and pepper in a bowl with the ground turkey. Roll the mixture into meatballs.

2. Using a pan over medium heat, preheat one tablespoon of olive oil. Add the meatballs and cook them until they're browned and cooked, which should take about 10 minutes. Set them aside.

3. Toss in the zucchini noodles after adding another spoonful of olive oil to the pan. Sauté them for about 2-3 minutes. You want them to be tender but still have a bit of a crunch.

4. Warm the marinara sauce in a pot or the microwave.

5. To serve, place a generous helping of zucchini noodles on each plate, top with the turkey meatballs, and spoon over the marinara sauce.

Nutritional Values (per serving):

- Calories: Approximately 350
- Protein: 27g
- Fat: 17g
- Carbohydrates: 20g
- Fiber: 4g

Cooking Time: About 30 minutes

Rating: ★★★★☆ (4/5) - It's a healthy and delicious twist on a classic!

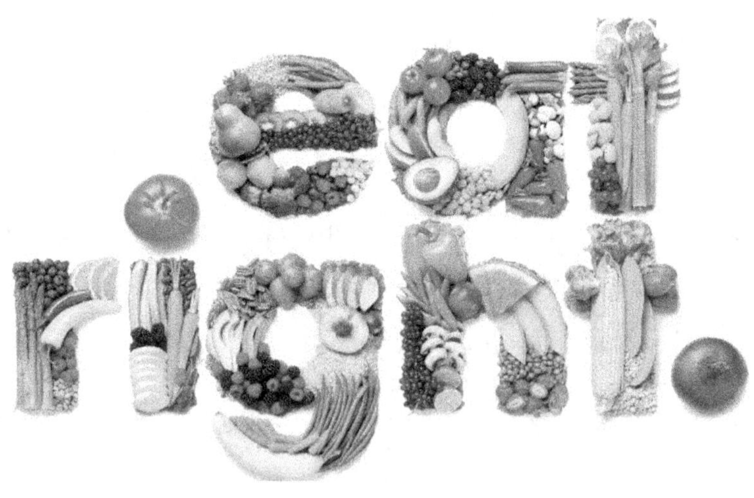

Snack and Sides

S nacks and sides are important but sometimes disregarded when it comes to gout management. The key to preventing gout flare-ups is including foods low in purines, which is made possible by these smaller meals. Consider whole grains, fresh produce, and fruits. Not only can they assist in maintaining reduced uric acid levels, but they also keep you full between meals. The secret is to choose sides and snacks that are as tasty as they are healthful for managing gout. In this manner, you're promoting your health and having fun with your food, which is crucial!

Carrot and Celery Sticks with Hummus

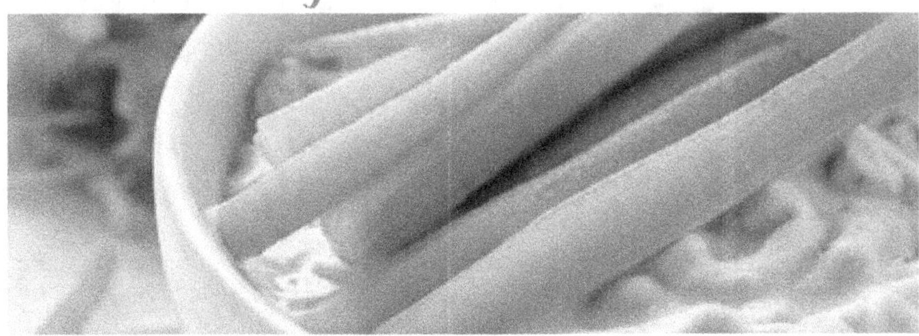

Ingredients:

- 2 large carrots
- 2 stalks of celery
- 1 cup of your favorite hummus (store-bought or homemade)

Preparation Steps:

1. This is as easy as it gets! Start by washing the carrots and celery thoroughly.

2. Peel the carrots and then chop both the carrots and celery into sticks. Aim for bite-size pieces that are easy to dip.

3. Scoop your hummus into a small bowl or divide it into individual serving containers if you're on the go.

4. That's it! Dip your veggie sticks into the hummus and enjoy.

Nutritional Values (per serving):

- Calories: About 150-200 (depending on the amount of hummus)
- Protein: 6g
- Fat: 12g (mostly healthy fats from the hummus)
- Carbohydrates: 10-15g
- Fiber: 5g

Cooking Time: About 5 minutes (just prep time)

Rating: ★★★★★ (5/5) - It's healthy, crunchy, and so easy to make!

Fresh Fruit Salad

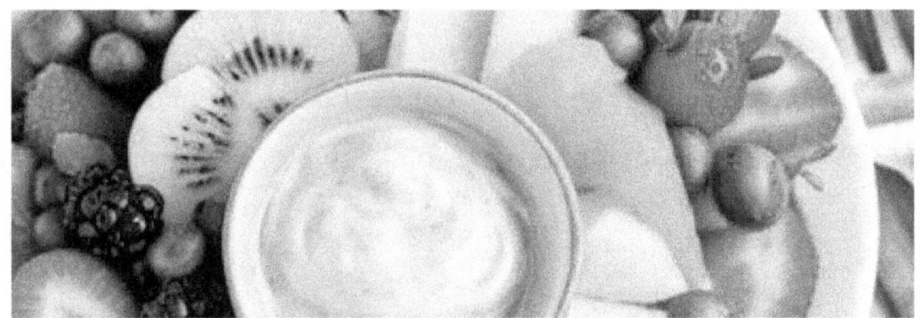

Ingredients:

- 1 cup strawberries, hulled and halved
- 1 cup blueberries
- 1 cup grapes (green or red)
- 1 banana, sliced
- 1 apple, cored and chopped
- 1 orange, peeled and sectioned
- Juice of 1 lemon
- Optional: a handful of chopped mint or a drizzle of honey for extra flavor

Preparation Steps:

1. This is as simple as prep can be. Start by washing all your fruits thoroughly.

2. Cut the strawberries, banana, apple, and orange into bite-sized pieces. Leave the blueberries and grapes whole.

3. Toss all the fruits into a large bowl. The more colorful, the better!

4. Squeeze the lemon juice over the fruits. This adds a zesty flavor and helps keep fruits like apples and bananas from browning.

5. Gently mix everything. If you're using mint or honey, now's the time to add them.

6. Put the fruit salad in the fridge for about an hour before serving. This step is optional, but it does make the salad extra refreshing.

Nutritional Values (per serving):

- Calories: About 100-150
- Protein: 1-2g
- Fat: Less than 1g
- Carbohydrates: 30-40g
- Fiber: 4-5g

Cooking Time: About 10 minutes (plus chilling time if you prefer)

Rating: ★★★★★ (5/5) - It's a delightful mix of sweet and tangy flavors!

Baked Sweet Potato Fries

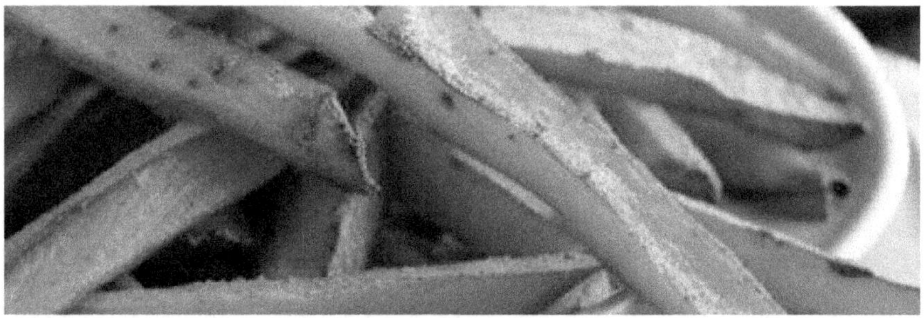

Ingredients:

- 2 large sweet potatoes
- 2 tablespoons olive oil
- Salt and pepper to taste
- Optional: a pinch of paprika or garlic powder for extra flavor

Preparation Steps:

1. Set your oven's temperature to 425°F (220°C) to begin. This high heat is key to getting those fries nice and crispy.

2. Wash and peel the sweet potatoes. Then cut them into fry-shaped sticks – try to keep them evenly sized so they cook uniformly.

3. Toss the sweet potato sticks in a big bowl with olive oil, salt, pepper, and any extra spices you choose. Make sure they're well coated.

4. Arrange the fries in a solitary layer on a baking sheet. It's important not to overcrowd them; they need space to get crispy.

5. Bake in the oven for about 20-25 minutes. Halfway through, flip the fries to get evenly crispy on all sides.

6. Once they're done, the fries should be golden and crispy on the outside and tender on the inside.

Nutritional Values (per serving):

- Calories: About 200
- Protein: 2g
- Fat: 7g
- Carbohydrates: 34g
- Fiber: 5g

Cooking Time: About 30-35 minutes

Rating: ★★★★★ (5/5) - They're a crowd-pleaser and a healthier alternative to regular fries!

Cucumber and Chickpea Salad

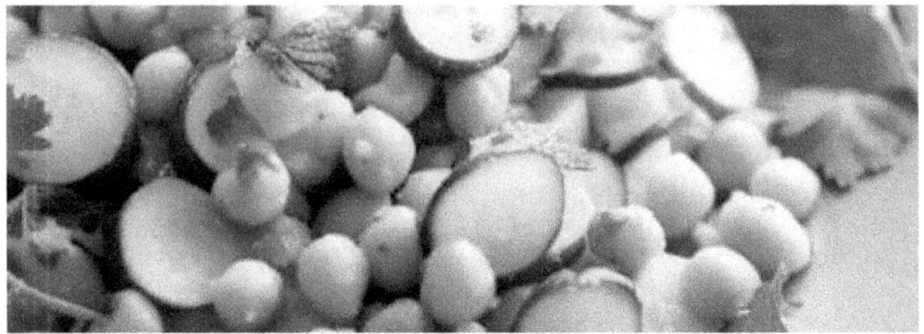

Ingredients:

- One can (15 oz) chickpeas, drained and rinsed
- 1 large cucumber, diced
- 1/4 red onion, thinly sliced
- 1/4 cup fresh parsley, chopped
- 2 tablespoons olive oil
- 1 tablespoon lemon juice
- 1 clove garlic, minced
- Salt and pepper to taste
- Optional: crumbled feta cheese or a sprinkle of paprika for extra flavor

Preparation Steps:

1. Combine the chickpeas, diced cucumber, sliced red onion, and chopped parsley in a bowl.

2. Mix the lemon juice, olive oil, minced garlic, salt, and minced garlic, and pepper in a small bowl or a jar to create your dressing.

3. Toss the salad with the dressing until everything is well-coated. The lemon juice will add a lovely zest, while the olive oil brings it all together.

4. For added taste, top with crumbled feta cheese or a sprinkle of paprika.

5. Let the salad sit briefly before serving, allowing the flavors to meld together beautifully.

Nutritional Values (per serving):

- Calories: Approximately 200
- Protein: 8g
- Fat: 9g
- Carbohydrates: 24g
- Fiber: 6g

Cooking Time: About 10 minutes (just prep time)

Rating: ★★★★★ (5/5) - It's fresh, healthy, and super easy to whip up!

Roasted Mixed Nuts

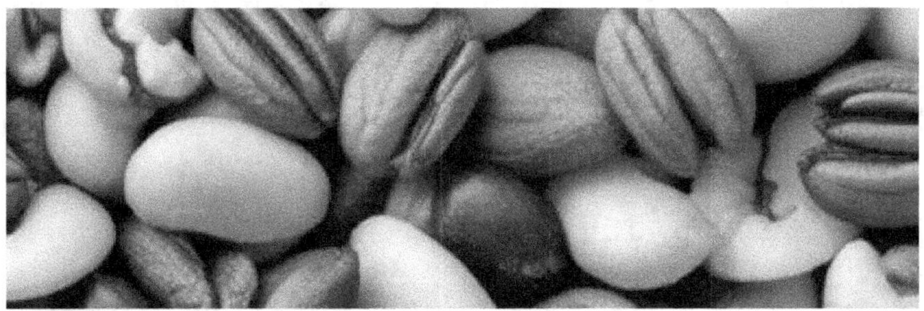

Ingredients:

- 2 cups mixed nuts (like almonds, walnuts, pecans, and cashews)
- 1 tablespoon olive oil
- 1 teaspoon sea salt

- Optional: a pinch of your favorite spices like paprika, garlic powder, or rosemary for extra flavor

Preparation Steps:

1. Preheat the oven to 350°F (175°C). It's all about that slow roast to bring out the nuts' natural flavors.

2. Toss the mixed nuts with olive oil and sea salt in a bowl. If you're using additional spices, add them at this stage.

3. On a baking sheet, arrange the nuts in a single layer. You want to give them space so they roast evenly.

4. Pop them in the oven and roast for about 10-15 minutes. Keep an eye on them and stir them halfway through to ensure they're roasting evenly.

5. Once they're golden and fragrant, take them out and let them cool. They'll get crunchier as they cool down.

Nutritional Values (per serving, about 1/4 cup):

- Calories: Approximately 200
- Protein: 5g
- Fat: 18g (mostly healthy fats)
- Carbohydrates: 6g
- Fiber: 3g

Cooking Time: About 20 minutes (including prep and roasting)

Rating: ★★★★★ (5/5) - They're a healthy, tasty, and versatile snack!

Fish and Seafoods

It might be a bit of a balancing act to manage gout while eating seafood and fish. There are many more fish alternatives that may be enjoyed in moderation, even if some seafood—like anchovies, mackerel, and shellfish—have a high purine content and should be avoided. In addition to having less purines, fish like tilapia, salmon, and trout are high in omega-3 fatty acids, which are excellent for general health. By including them into your diet, you may maintain a gout-friendly eating plan while also adding tasty diversity and vital minerals. Recall that it all comes down to making wise decisions and taking use of the sea's riches in a way that advances your health objectives!

Baked Cod with Lemon and Dill

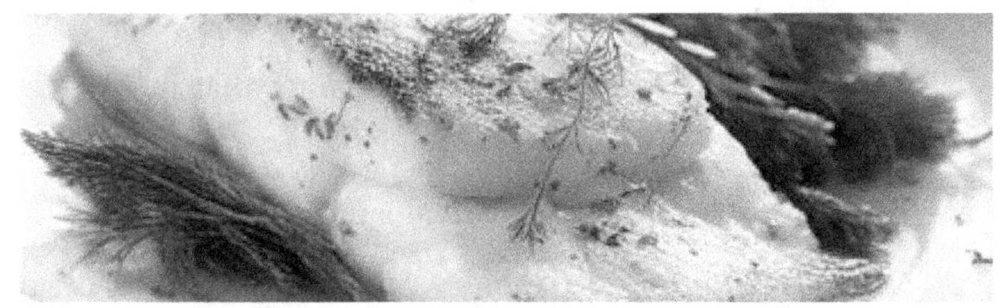

Ingredients:

- 4 cod fillets (about 6 ounces each)
- 2 tablespoons olive oil
- 1 lemon, thinly sliced
- 2 tablespoons fresh dill, chopped
- Salt and pepper to taste
- Optional: a sprinkle of garlic powder or paprika for extra flavor

Preparation Steps:

1. Preheat your oven to 400 degrees Fahrenheit (200 degrees Celsius). This temperature is ideal for evenly and speedily roasting the fish.
2. To prevent the fish from sticking, lightly oil a baking dish with 1 tablespoon olive oil.
3. Arrange the fish fillets in a plate. Drizzle the remaining olive oil over them and season with salt, pepper, and any other spices you're using.
4. Garnish each fillet with lemon slices and plenty of fresh dill. As the fish bakes, the lemon will infuse it with a beautiful citrus taste.
5. Bake the fish for 12-15 minutes, or until it flakes easily with a fork. The precise duration will depend on the thickness of your fillets.
6. When finished, set aside for a few minutes before serving.

Nutritional Values (per serving):

- Calories: About 200
- Protein: 30g
- Fat: 8g (mostly healthy fats from the olive oil)

- Carbohydrates: 1g
- Fiber: 0g

Cooking Time: About 20 minutes

Rating: ★★★★★ (5/5) - It's a simple, elegant, and healthy dish!

Shrimp and Avocado Salad

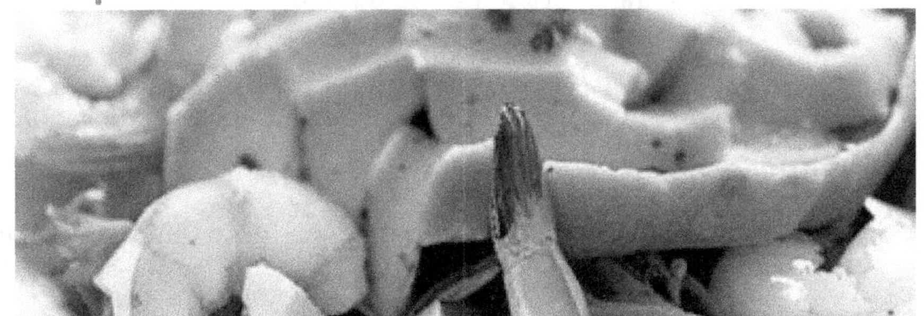

Ingredients:

- 1-pound large shrimp, peeled and deveined
- 2 ripe avocados, diced
- 1 cup cherry tomatoes, halved
- 1 cucumber, diced
- 1/4 red onion, finely chopped

- 2 tablespoons fresh cilantro or parsley, chopped
- 2 tablespoons olive oil
- Juice of 1 lime
- 1 clove garlic, minced
- Salt and pepper to taste

- Optional: a pinch of chili flakes for some heat

Preparation Steps:

1. Begin by preparing the shrimp. To achieve the same color and consistency, you may sauté them in a skillet with a little olive oil or boil them in salted water for two to three minutes. Give them time to cool.
2. Put the diced avocados, cherry tomatoes, cucumber, red onion, and chopped parsley or cilantro in a big bowl.
3. Fill the dish with the cooked shrimp.
4. Combine the olive oil, lime juice, minced garlic, salt, pepper, and chili flakes (if using) in another small bowl.
5. Lightly mix everything to coat after drizzling the salad components with the dressing.
6. Taste it and, if necessary, adjust the seasoning.

Nutritional Values (per serving):

- Calories: About 350
- Protein: 25g
- Fat: 20g (mostly healthy fats from the avocado and olive oil)
- Carbohydrates: 20g
- Fiber: 9g

Cooking Time: About 15-20 minutes

Rating: ★★★★★ (5/5) - It's a refreshing and satisfying salad!

Grilled Tilapia with Mango Salsa

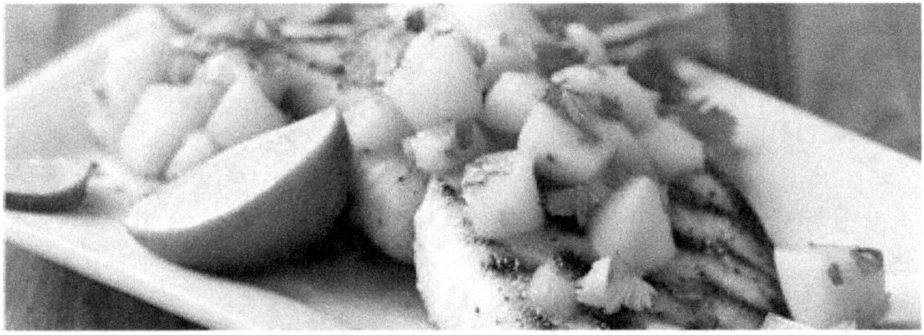

Ingredients: For the Grilled Tilapia:

- 4 tilapia fillets (about 6 ounces each)
- 2 tablespoons olive oil
- 1 teaspoon paprika
- 1/2 teaspoon cumin
- Salt and pepper to taste
- For the Mango Salsa:
- 2 ripe mangos, peeled and diced
- 1 red bell pepper, diced
- 1/4 red onion, finely chopped
- 1/4 cup fresh cilantro, chopped
- Juice of 1 lime
- Salt and pepper to taste
- Optional: a pinch of chili flakes for some heat

Preparation Steps: For the Grilled Tilapia:

1. Turn the heat up to medium-high on your grill. The tilapia may alternatively be baked or cooked in a grill pan.
2. To make a tasty marinade, combine the olive oil, paprika, cumin, salt, and pepper in a small bowl.

3. Apply the marinade to the tilapia fillets on both sides.

4. Grill the tilapia until it flakes easily with a fork, about 3 to 4 minutes on each side. Depending on the thickness of the fillets, the precise duration may change.

For the Mango Salsa:

1. Put the chopped red onion, cilantro, red bell pepper, and diced mango in a basin.

2. Drizzle the mixture with one lime juice.

3. If you enjoy a little heat, season with chili flakes, salt, and pepper.

4. Now that your mango salsa is ready, give it a nice toss.

Nutritional Values (per serving):

- Calories: About 250
- Protein: 30g
- Fat: 8g (mostly healthy fats from the olive oil)
- Carbohydrates: 20g
- Fiber: 3g

Cooking Time: About 20 minutes

Rating: ★★★★★ (5/5) - It's a tropical delight on your plate!

Seafood Paella with Brown Rice

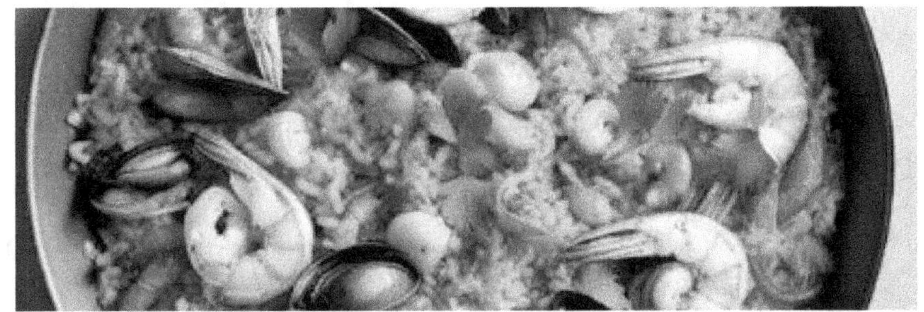

Ingredients:

- 1 cup brown rice

- 1/2-pound large shrimp, peeled and deveined

- 1/2-pound mussels, cleaned and debearded

- 1/2-pound clams, cleaned

- 1/2-pound firm white fish (such as cod or halibut), cut into chunks

- 2 tablespoons olive oil

- 1 onion, finely chopped

- 1 red bell pepper, diced

- 2 cloves garlic, minced

- 1 teaspoon smoked paprika

- 1/2 teaspoon saffron threads (optional, but adds a wonderful flavor and color)

- 1/2 teaspoon cayenne pepper (adjust to your spice preference)

- 1 can (14 oz) diced tomatoes

- 2 cups chicken or vegetable broth

- 1/2 cup frozen peas

- Salt and pepper to taste
- Fresh parsley for garnish
- Lemon wedges for garnish

Preparation Steps:

1. Begin by cooking the brown rice as directed on the packet. It should be somewhat firm yet still delicate. Put it away.

2. Heat the olive oil in a wide skillet or a sizable paella pan over medium heat.

3. Include the minced garlic, diced red bell pepper, and chopped onion. Cook them until they are aromatic and tender.

4. Stir in the smoked paprika, saffron threads (if using), and cayenne pepper. This is when the flavors of paella start to work their magic!

5. Add the chopped tomatoes along with their liquid and heat until they begin to soften, maybe a few minutes.

6. Add the brown rice and stir to coat it in the tomato sauce.

7. Add the broth (either chicken or veggie) and boil. Give it a good 10 minutes to simmer so the flavors can combine.

8. Carefully place the seafood—white fish, mussels, clams, and shrimp—atop the rice mixture.

9. Once the seafood is fully cooked, cover the pan and simmer for an additional 10 to 15 minutes. The shrimp and fish should become opaque, and the mussels and clams should open.

10. Add the frozen peas and simmer for a further two to three minutes, or until well cooked.

11. Season to taste with salt and pepper.

12. Add some fresh parsley and lemon wedges as garnish.

Nutritional Values (per serving):

- Calories: About 400-450

- Carbohydrates: 50g

- Protein: 30g

- Fiber: 6g

- Fat: 10g (mostly healthy fats from the olive oil and seafood)

Cooking Time: About 45-50 minutes

Rating: ★★★★★ (5/5) - It's a Spanish masterpiece that's worth the effort!

Teriyaki Glazed Salmon

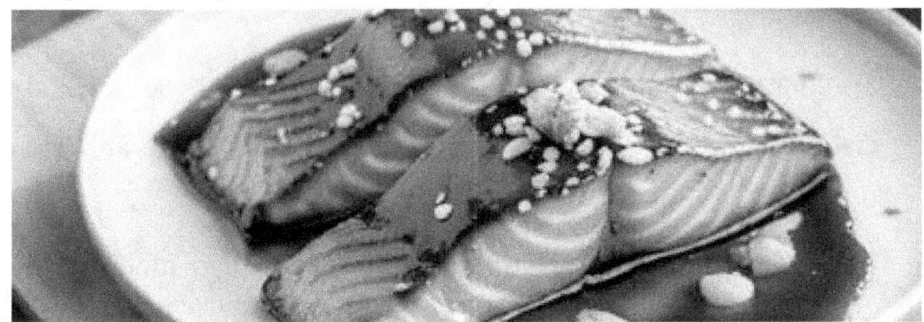

Ingredients:

- 4 salmon fillets (about 6 ounces each)

- 1/2 cup teriyaki sauce (store-bought or homemade)

- 2 tablespoons soy sauce

- 2 tablespoons brown sugar

- 2 cloves garlic, minced

- 1 teaspoon ginger, grated (fresh or powdered)

- Optional: sesame seeds and chopped green onions for garnish

Preparation Steps:

1. Combine the brown sugar, soy sauce, teriyaki sauce, grated ginger, and chopped garlic in a bowl. This produces a marinade with taste.

2. Transfer the salmon fillets to a plastic bag that can be sealed or a shallow plate.

3. Evenly cover each fillet of salmon with the marinade, being sure to do so.

4. To enable the salmon to marinade and absorb those delectable tastes, seal the dish or bag and place it in the refrigerator for at least half an hour.

5. Use a stovetop grill pan or preheat your grill to medium-high heat.

6. Remove the salmon from the marinade and cook for about 4-5 minutes on each side, or until the salmon flakes easily with a fork. As it cooks, brush with the marinade that was set aside.

7. If you would rather bake the salmon in the oven, roast it for 15 to 20 minutes at 400°F (200°C), basting it periodically with marinade.

8. To enhance taste and appearance, sprinkle chopped green onions and sesame seeds on top after cooking.

Nutritional Values (per serving):

- Calories: About 300-350
- Protein: 30g
- Fat: 12g (healthy fats from the salmon)
- Carbohydrates: 20g
- Fiber: 0g

Cooking Time: About 30-40 minutes (including marinating time)

Rating: ★★★★★ (5/5) - It's a savory delight that's both easy and delicious!

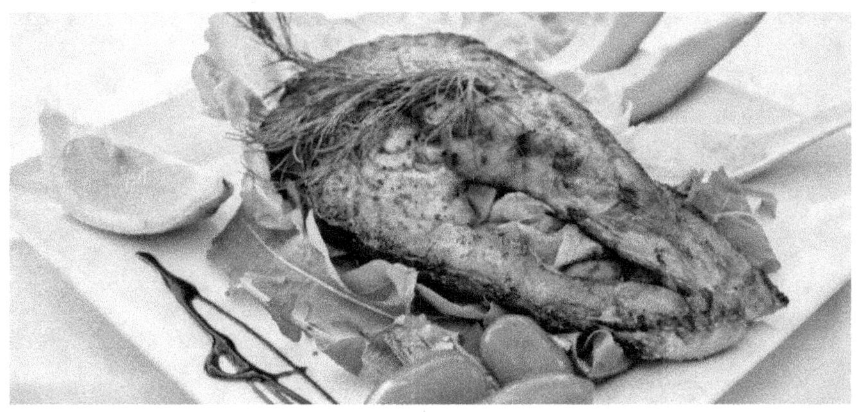

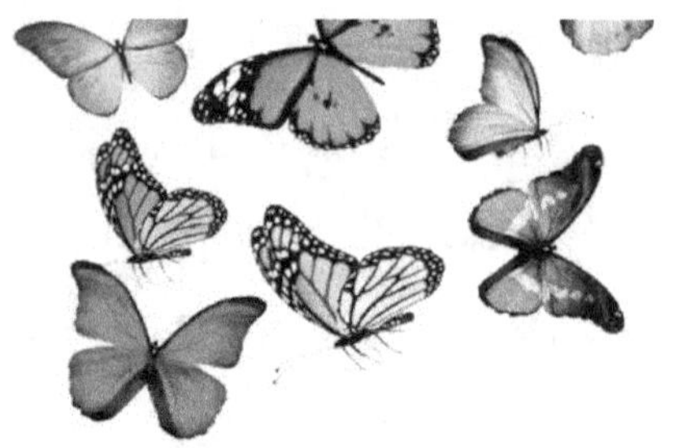

"Your decision to manage gout through nutrition is a powerful step towards better health. Every nutritious meal is a step forward in this journey. Remember, small changes can lead to big victories. Keep focusing on eating wholesome foods that nourish your body and reduce inflammation. Your dedication and commitment are inspiring. You're not just fighting gout; you're embracing a healthier, happier life. Stay motivated and strong!"

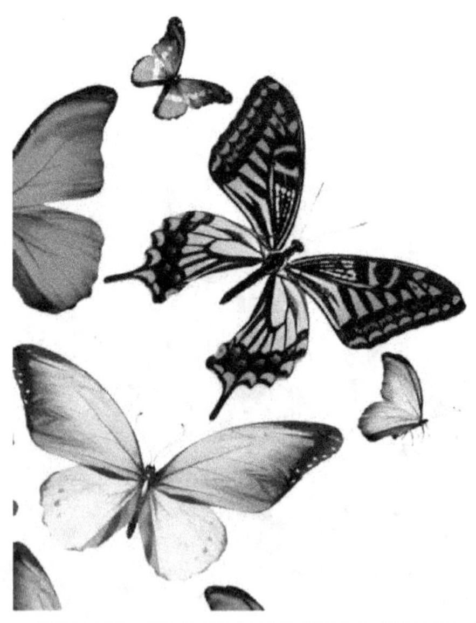

Chicken Recipes

Chicken meals may be a delightful and healthful option for gout management. Compared to certain other meats, chicken is a lean protein source with less purines. This makes it a fantastic choice for people who want to eat delectable food and manage their gout. A gout-friendly diet can include a variety of chicken recipes, such as delicious stir-fries or grilled chicken. Now let's explore some delicious and thoughtful ways to eat chicken that can help you achieve your gout treatment objectives!

Chicken and Vegetable Kabobs

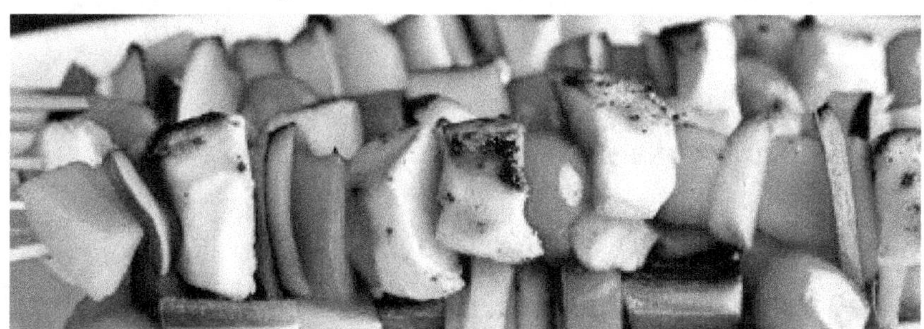

Ingredients:

- 1-pound boneless, skinless chicken breasts, cut into chunks
- 2 bell peppers (red, green, or yellow), cut into chunks
- 1 red onion, cut into chunks
- 1 zucchini, sliced into rounds
- 8-10 wooden skewers (pre-soaked in water for about 30 minutes to prevent burning)
- 2 tablespoons olive oil
- 2 cloves garlic, minced
- 1 teaspoon dried oregano
- Juice of 1 lemon
- Salt and pepper to taste
- Optional: cherry tomatoes, mushrooms, or other favorite veggies for a variety

Preparation Steps:

1. Combine the olive oil, lemon juice, dried oregano, minced garlic, salt, and pepper in a bowl. This produces a marinade with taste.

2. After submerging the chicken chunks in the marinade, let them sit for at least 20 to 30 minutes so they can absorb the flavor. They can be marinated in the refrigerator.

3. Assemble your kabobs by skewering bell peppers, zucchini, red onions, chicken, and any additional vegetables you like in that order.

4. Turn the heat up to medium-high on your grill.

5. Grill the kabobs for ten to fifteen minutes, rotating them now and again, or until the chicken is well cooked and the vegetables are soft and slightly browned.

6. For added flavor, spread any remaining marinade over the kabobs while they're cooking.

Nutritional Values (per serving, approximately 2 kabobs):

- Calories: About 250-300
- Protein: 25g
- Fat: 8g (mostly healthy fats from the olive oil and chicken)
- Carbohydrates: 20g
- Fiber: 4g

Cooking Time: About 25-30 minutes (including marinating time)

Rating: ★★★★★ (5/5) - It's a tasty and fun meal for everyone!

Lemon Herb Roasted Chicken

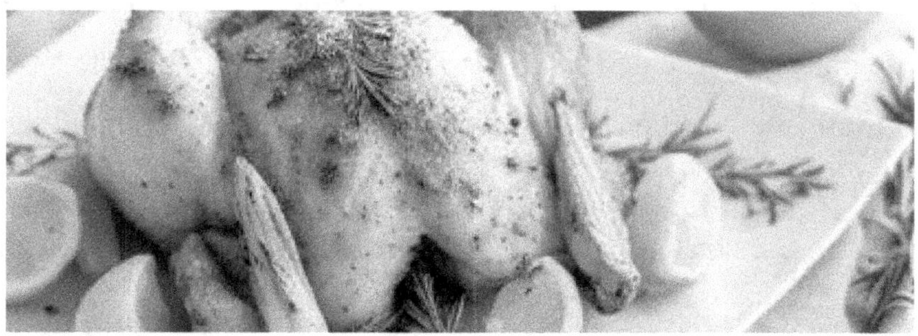

Ingredients:

- 1 whole chicken (about 4-5 pounds)
- 2 lemons, one sliced and one juiced
- 4-6 cloves garlic, minced
- 2 tablespoons olive oil
- 2 teaspoons dried thyme
- 2 teaspoons dried rosemary
- Salt and pepper to taste
- Optional: fresh herbs like rosemary and thyme sprigs for garnish

Preparation Steps:

1. Set the oven temperature to 375°F or 190°C.
2. Rinse the chicken from top to bottom and use paper towels to pat dry. This aids in roasting skin that is crispy.
3. Liberally season the chicken on the outside as well as the interior with salt and pepper.
4. Combine the minced garlic, dried thyme, dried rosemary, and lemon juice in a small bowl.
5. Carefully peel the chicken's skin and smear the combination of herbs and garlic under it. This infuses the meat with taste.
6. Stuff the chicken's cavity with the lemon slices and any remaining herb mixture.
7. To ensure consistent cooking, tie the chicken legs together using kitchen thread.
8. To give the chicken a gorgeous golden hue, brush it with olive oil.
9. Put the bird, breast-side up, in a roasting pan.

10. Roast the chicken for one hour and fifteen minutes to one hour and thirty minutes, or until its internal temperature reaches 165°F (74°C), in a preheated oven.

11. For an elegant appearance, you may optionally add fresh thyme and rosemary sprigs as a garnish.

Nutritional Values (per serving, about 1/4 chicken):

- Calories: About 300-350
- Protein: 30g
- Fat: 20g (mostly from the chicken skin)
- Carbohydrates: 3g
- Fiber: 1g

Cooking Time: About 1 hour and 30 minutes

Rating: ★★★★★ (5/5) - It's a timeless and delicious favorite!

Chicken Caesar Salad with Low-Fat Dressing

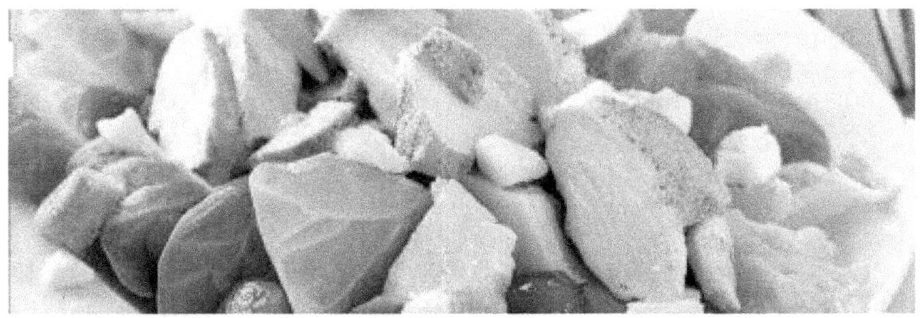

Ingredients: For the Salad:

- 2 boneless, skinless chicken breasts
- 1 head of romaine lettuce, chopped

- 1 cup whole wheat croutons (store-bought or homemade)
- Grated Parmesan cheese for garnish
- Lemon wedges for garnish (optional)

For the Low-Fat Caesar Dressing:

- 1/2 cup Greek yogurt (plain, non-fat)

- 2 tablespoons light mayonnaise
- 2 cloves garlic, minced
- 2 tablespoons grated Parmesan cheese
- 2 teaspoons Dijon mustard
- 2 teaspoons Worcestershire sauce
- Juice of 1 lemon
- Salt and pepper to taste

Preparation Steps: For the Chicken:

1. Use salt and pepper to season the chicken breasts.
2. Add the chicken to a hot grill or grill pan and cook it for 6–7 minutes on each side, or until it's cooked through. Slice into strips after letting it rest for a few minutes.

For the Caesar Dressing with Low Fat:

1. In a bowl, mix the Greek yogurt, light mayonnaise, chopped garlic, grated Parmesan cheese, Dijon mustard, Worcestershire sauce, lemon juice, salt, and pepper. This produces your fat-free, creamy Caesar dressing.

For Putting the Salad Together:

1. Combine the dressing and chopped romaine lettuce in a large salad dish, tossing to coat completely.

2. Include the whole wheat croutons and the grilled chicken strips.

3. Combine everything until the salad has an even dressing and well-combined components.

4. If you want to add a little zing, garnish with lemon slices and grated Parmesan cheese.

Nutritional Values (per serving):

- Calories: About 350-400
- Protein: 30g
- Fat: 10g (mostly from the chicken and low-fat dressing)
- Carbohydrates: 35g
- Fiber: 5g

Cooking Time: About 20-25 minutes

Rating: ★★★★★ (5/5) - It's a healthy and delicious salad!

Chicken and Broccoli Stir-Fry

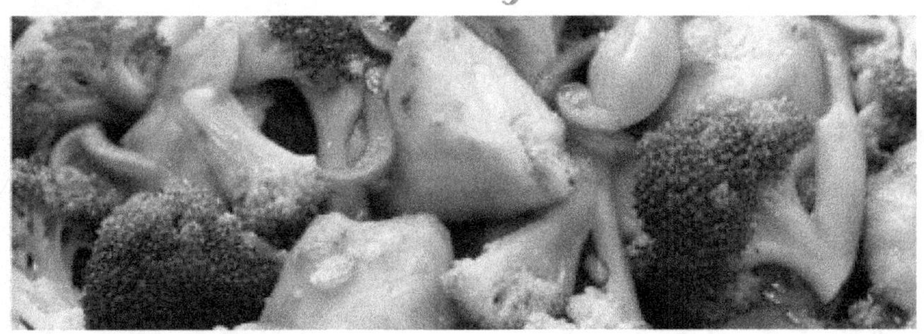

Ingredients: For the Stir-Fry:

- 2 boneless, skinless chicken breasts, cut into bite-sized pieces
- 1 head of broccoli, cut into florets
- 2 cloves garlic, minced
- 1 tablespoon vegetable oil (such as canola or peanut oil)
- Optional: sliced bell peppers, carrots, or snap peas for extra veggies

For the Stir-Fry Sauce:

- 1/4 cup low-sodium soy sauce
- 2 tablespoons hoisin sauce
- 1 tablespoon honey
- 1 teaspoon sesame oil
- 1 teaspoon cornstarch (to thicken the sauce)
- Red pepper flakes (optional, for a bit of heat)

Preparation Steps:

1. Combine the soy sauce, hoisin sauce, honey, sesame oil, cornstarch, and red pepper flakes (if using) in a small dish to make the stir-fry sauce. Put this sauce away.
2. In a large skillet or wok, heat the vegetable oil over medium-high heat.
3. Add the minced garlic and stir until fragrant, about 30 seconds.
4. When the chicken pieces are cooked through and beginning to brown, add them to the skillet and stir-fry for five to six minutes. After removing it from the pan, set the chicken aside.

5. Stir-fry the broccoli and any other vegetables you're using in the same skillet for approximately 4–5 minutes, or until they're crisp but still soft. Add a little extra oil if necessary.

6. Add the cooked chicken and broccoli back to the skillet.

7. Drizzle the chicken and broccoli with the stir-fried sauce.

8. Cook, stirring, for a further two to three minutes, or until the sauce thickens and covers the ingredients.

9. If preferred, serve the hot stir-fry over prepared rice or noodles.

Nutritional Values (per serving, excluding rice or noodles):

- Calories: About 300-350
- Protein: 30g
- Fat: 10g (mostly from cooking oil)
- Carbohydrates: 20g
- Fiber: 4g

Cooking Time: About 20-25 minutes

Rating: ★★★★★ (5/5) - It's a quick and tasty weeknight dinner!

Grilled Chicken Caesar Wraps

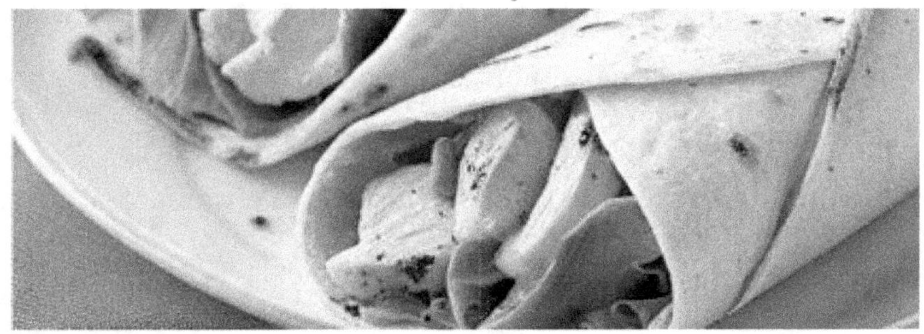

Ingredients: For the Grilled Chicken:

- 2 boneless, skinless chicken breasts
- 1 tablespoon olive oil
- Salt and pepper to taste
- 1 teaspoon dried oregano (optional, for extra flavor)

For the Caesar Dressing:

- 1/2 cup Caesar dressing (store-bought or homemade)
- Juice of 1 lemon
- 1/4 cup grated Parmesan cheese

For the Wraps:

- 4 large whole wheat or spinach tortillas
- 2 cups chopped romaine lettuce
- 1/2 cup croutons
- Additional grated Parmesan cheese for garnish
- Optional: cherry tomatoes, sliced cucumbers, or any other favorite salad ingredients

Preparation Steps: For the Grilled Chicken:

1. Add dried oregano, salt, and pepper to the chicken breasts.
2. Turn the heat up to medium-high on a grill or grill pan.
3. Coat the chicken with olive oil and place it on the grill for 6–7 minutes on each side, or until it is cooked through and has a hint of charring.
4. Before slicing the chicken into strips, let it a few minutes to rest.

Regarding the Caesar Dressing:

1. Combine the grated Parmesan cheese, lemon juice, and Caesar dressing in a bowl. This produces your creamy Caesar dressing.

For Putting the Wraps Together:

1. Arrange the tortillas on a sanitized surface.
2. Evenly distribute a little Caesar dressing over each tortilla.
3. Top each tortilla with a little bit of chopped romaine lettuce.
4. Add croutons and fried chicken pieces on top.
5. You may optionally add sliced cucumbers, cherry tomatoes, or any other salad elements you choose.
6. For added taste, add a little more grated Parmesan cheese.
7. To make a wrap, fold the tortilla in half lengthwise and roll it securely.

Nutritional Values (per wrap):

- Calories: About 350-400
- Protein: 25g
- Fat: 20g (mostly from the Caesar dressing and chicken)
- Carbohydrates: 25g
- Fiber: 4g

Preparation Time: About 20-25 minutes

Rating: ★★★★★ (5/5) - It's a tasty and convenient meal!

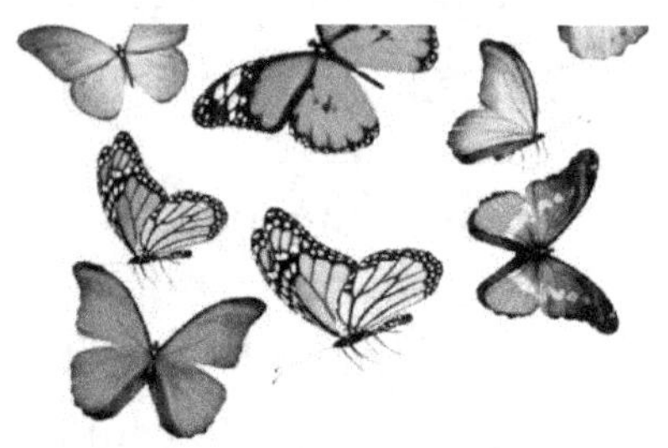

"Tackling gout with a nutritional approach is a testament to your strength and determination. Each healthy meal is a building block in your path to wellness. Focus on the vibrant colors and natural flavors of fruits, vegetables, and whole grains. They're your allies in this fight. Celebrate each day of progress, no matter how small. Your journey is about progress, not perfection. Keep going, you're doing great!"

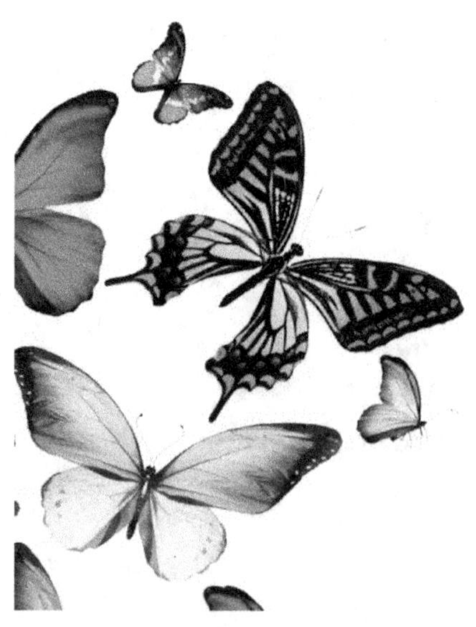

Beef and Pork Recipes

If chosen and cooked carefully, meals including beef and pork may be tasty solutions for treating gout. These meats may add taste and protein to your meals, but you should always choose lean cuts and watch how much you eat. You may enjoy beef and pig meals that support your gout management objectives by making the appropriate food selections and cooking methods. Let's look at some delicious and health-conscious meals that include these meats and are suitable for gout treatment!

Grilled Lean Beef Burgers with Whole Grain Buns

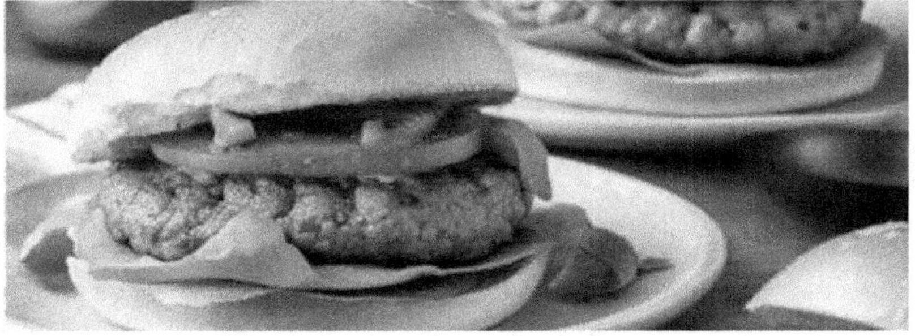

Ingredients: For the Beef Patties:

- 1-pound lean ground beef (at least 90% lean)
- 1/4 cup finely chopped onions
- 1 clove garlic, minced
- Salt and pepper to taste
- Optional: a pinch of smoked paprika for extra flavor

For the Burger Assembly:

- 4 whole grain burger buns
- Lettuce leaves
- Tomato slices
- Onion rings
- Pickles
- Mustard and ketchup (optional)
- Cheese slices (optional)

Preparation Steps: For the Beef Patties:

1. Put the lean ground beef, minced garlic, finely chopped onions, salt, pepper, and smoky paprika (if using) in a bowl.
2. Gently combine the ingredients, taking care not to overwork the meat.
3. Create four equal parts out of the mixture, then form them into burger patties.

To Grill:

1. Turn the heat up to medium-high on your grill.
2. Transfer the burger patties to the grill and cook for 3–4 minutes on each side, or until cooked through to your preferred consistency.

3. If you want to add cheese, put a piece on each burger and let it melt in the last minute of cooking.

4. You can also toast the whole grain burger buns on the grill while the patties are cooking.

For Putting the Burgers Together:

1. Arrange a leaf of lettuce on the lower portion of every bun.

2. Include a burger patty, cheese included or not.

3. Add pickles, tomato slices, and onion rings on top.

4. For added taste, feel free to add ketchup and mustard.

5. Use the upper portion of the whole-grain bun to finish.

Nutritional Values (per burger):

- Calories: About 300-350
- Protein: 25g
- Fat: 10g (mostly from the lean beef)
- Carbohydrates: 30g
- Fiber: 5g

Cooking Time: About 10-15 minutes

Rating: ★★★★★ (5/5) - It's a satisfying and wholesome burger!

Stir-fried pork with Bell Peppers and Snow Peas

Ingredients: For the Stir-Fry:

- 1 pound pork tenderloin, thinly sliced into strips
- 1 red bell pepper, sliced

- 1 yellow bell pepper, sliced
- 1 cup snow peas, trimmed
- 2 cloves garlic, minced
- 2 tablespoons vegetable oil (such as canola or peanut oil)
- Optional: sliced onions or carrots for added veggies

For the Stir-Fry Sauce:

- 1/4 cup low-sodium soy sauce
- 2 tablespoons oyster sauce
- 1 tablespoon honey
- 1 teaspoon cornstarch (to thicken the sauce)
- Red pepper flakes (optional, for a bit of heat)

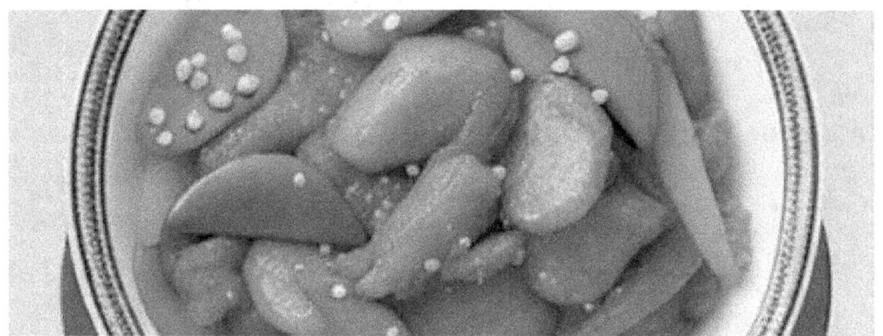

Preparation Steps: For the Stir-Fry:

1. Heat the vegetable oil in a big pan or wok over medium-high heat.

2. Stir-fry the minced garlic for about 30 seconds, or until aromatic.

3. When the pork is cooked through and beginning to brown, add the thinly sliced pork and stir-fry it for three to four minutes. After taking the meat out of the skillet, set it aside.

4. Add a little extra oil to the same skillet if necessary, and stir-fry the bell peppers, snow peas, and any other vegetables for three to four minutes, or until they are crisp but still soft.

5. Add the cooked pork and vegetables back to the skillet.

For the Sauce (Surfy):

1. Combine the honey, cornstarch, soy sauce, oyster sauce, and red pepper flakes (if using) in a bowl. This generates your flavorful stir-fry sauce.

To Complete the Plate:

1. Cover the pork and vegetables in the skillet with the stir-fry sauce.
2. Cook, stirring, for a further two to three minutes, or until the sauce thickens and covers the ingredients.
3. If preferred, serve the hot stir-fry over prepared rice or noodles.

Nutritional Values (per serving, excluding rice or noodles):

- Calories: About 300-350
- Protein: 25g
- Fat: 10g (mostly from cooking oil)
- Carbohydrates: 20g
- Fiber: 4g

Cooking Time: About 20-25 minutes

Rating: ★★★★★ (5/5) - It's a delicious and colorful stir-fry!

Beef and Vegetable Stew

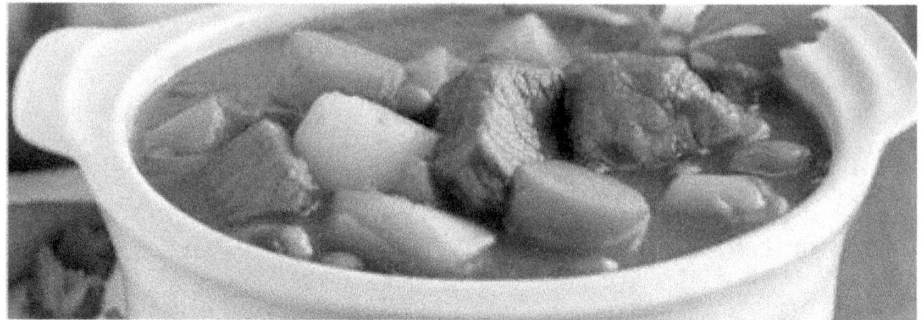

Ingredients:

- 1-pound lean beef stew meat, cut into cubes
- 2 tablespoons olive oil
- 1 onion, chopped
- 2 cloves garlic, minced
- 2 carrots, sliced
- 2 potatoes, diced
- 1 cup green beans, trimmed and cut into bite-sized pieces
- 4 cups beef broth (low-sodium)
- 1 can (14 ounces) diced tomatoes
- 1 teaspoon dried thyme
- 1 teaspoon dried rosemary
- Salt and pepper to taste
- Optional: a handful of chopped fresh parsley for garnish

Preparation Steps:

1. In a large saucepan or Dutch oven, heat the olive oil over medium-high heat.

2. Include the minced garlic and diced onion. Sauté for two to three minutes, or until the onion becomes transparent and aromatic.

3. Add the cubed meat and brown it on all sides for about 5-6 minutes.
4. Add the green beans, potatoes, and carrots and stir.
5. Add the diced tomatoes and their juices to the beef broth.
6. Include the rosemary and dried thyme. To taste, add salt and pepper for seasoning.
7. After bringing the mixture to a boil, lower the heat to a simmer, cover the pot, and let it there for one to two hours, or until the veggies are fully cooked and the meat is soft.
8. Before serving, you can choose to garnish with freshly chopped parsley.

Nutritional Values (per serving):

- Calories: About 350-400
- Protein: 25g
- Fat: 10g (mostly from the olive oil and beef)
- Carbohydrates: 30g
- Fiber: 5g

Cooking Time: About 2 hours (simmering time)

Rating: ★★★★★ (5/5) - It's a comforting and nourishing stew!

Pork Tenderloin with Apple Sauce

Ingredients: For the Pork Tenderloin:

- 1 pork tenderloin (about 1 pound)
- 1 tablespoon olive oil
- Salt and pepper to taste

- Optional: dried sage or rosemary for seasoning

For the Apple Sauce:

- 2-3 apples (such as Granny Smith or Fuji), peeled, cored, and chopped

- 1/4 cup water

- 2 tablespoons honey or brown sugar (adjust to taste)

- 1/2 teaspoon ground cinnamon

- 1/4 teaspoon ground nutmeg

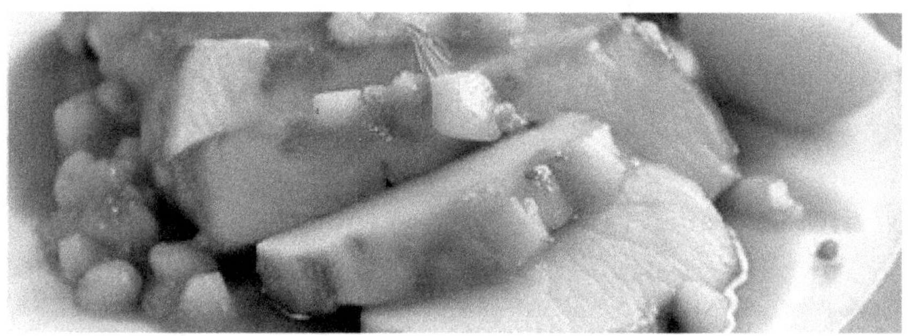

Preparation Steps: For the Pork Tenderloin:

2. Set the oven temperature to 375°F or 190°C.

3. Add salt, pepper, and, if preferred, dried sage or rosemary to the pork tenderloin's seasoning.

4. Heat the olive oil in a pan that is oven-safe over medium-high heat.

5. Add the pork tenderloin and sear it until it has a lovely brown color on all sides.

6. Place the skillet in the oven that has been warmed, and roast the pig for 15 to 20 minutes, or until its internal temperature reaches 145°F (63°C).
7. Before slicing the pork into medallions, take it out of the oven and let it a few minutes to rest.

Regarding the Apple Sauce:

1. You may make the apple sauce as the pork roasts.
2. Put the diced apples, water, honey (or brown sugar), powdered nutmeg, and cinnamon in a pot.
3. Simmer for ten to fifteen minutes, stirring now and again, over medium heat, or until the apples are tender and the sauce has thickened. You may taste and adjust the sweetness.
4. After the sauce is cooked, you may purée it until it's smooth using a blender or immersion blender.

Nutritional Values (per serving, including apple sauce):

- Calories: About 300-350
- Protein: 25g
- Fat: 10g (mostly from the pork)
- Carbohydrates: 30g
- Fiber: 4g

Cooking Time: About 30-35 minutes

Rating: ★★★★★ (5/5) - It's a flavorful and comforting meal!

Lean Beef Fajitas

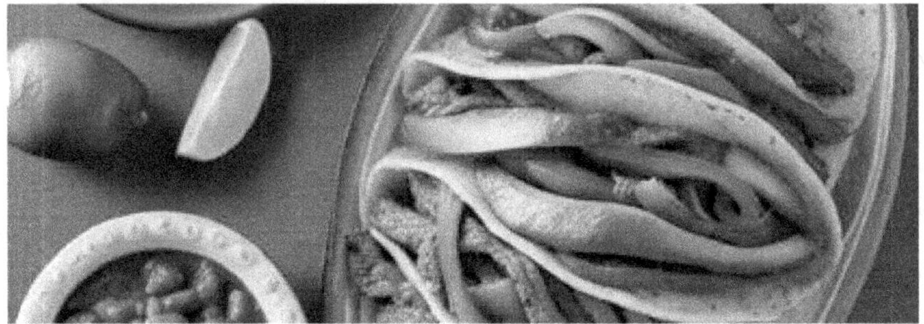

Ingredients: For the Beef Marinade:

- 1-pound lean beef (such as sirloin or flank steak), thinly sliced
- 2 cloves garlic, minced
- Juice of 2 limes
- 1 tablespoon olive oil
- 1 teaspoon ground cumin
- 1 teaspoon chili powder
- Salt and pepper to taste

For the Fajitas:

- 2 bell peppers (any color), thinly sliced
- 1 onion, thinly sliced
- 1 tablespoon vegetable oil (such as canola or peanut oil)
- 8 small whole wheat tortillas
- Optional toppings: salsa, guacamole, sour cream, shredded cheese, chopped cilantro, and lime wedges

Preparation Steps: For the Beef Marinade:

1. Combine the ground cumin, chili powder, lime juice, olive oil, chopped garlic, salt, and pepper in a bowl.

2. Transfer the thinly sliced beef to a shallow dish or zip-top bag, then cover it with the marinade. Refrigerate for a minimum of half an hour (or more if you have time) after sealing the bag or covering the dish.

Regarding the Fajitas:

1. Heat the vegetable oil in a large skillet or pan over medium-high heat.
2. Add the onions and bell peppers that have been cut to the skillet and cook for 4–5 minutes, or until they are soft and starting to caramelize. After taking them out of the skillet, set them aside.
3. Place the marinated beef slices in the same skillet and cook for 2 to 3 minutes on each side, or until cooked through to your preferred doneness.
4. You may reheat the tortillas in the oven or on a dry griddle while the meat cooks.
5. After the steak is done, add the onions and bell peppers that you sautéed back to the skillet and give everything a quick stir to reheat for approximately a minute.

Nutritional Values (per serving, including tortillas):

- Calories: About 350-400
- Protein: 25g
- Fat: 10g (mostly from the beef and vegetable oil)
- Carbohydrates: 30g
- Fiber: 4g

Cooking Time: About 20-25 minutes (including marinating time)

Rating: ★★★★★ (5/5) - It's a delicious and colorful Tex-Mex favorite!

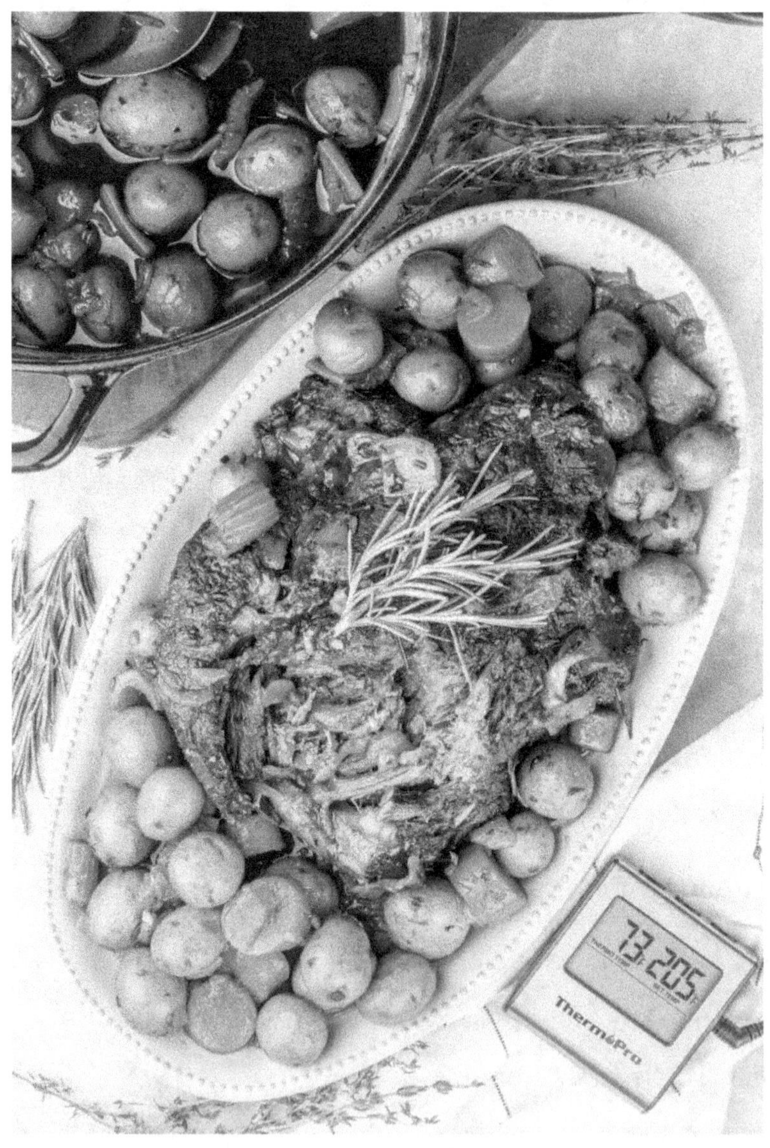

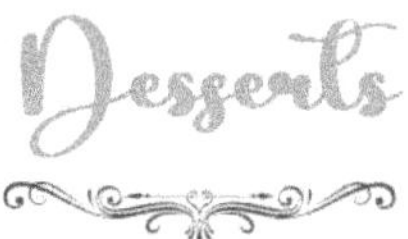

Desserts

Sweet treats don't have to be off-limits when it comes to managing gout. You may enjoy sweet snacks that fit within your gout-friendly diet if you make the appropriate choices. Desserts may be thoughtful and tasty, providing delight without making flare-ups of gout worse. Let's look at some delicious dessert ideas that go well with your gout treatment plan so you may indulge in life's sweeter side while still taking good care of your health.

Baked Apples with Cinnamon

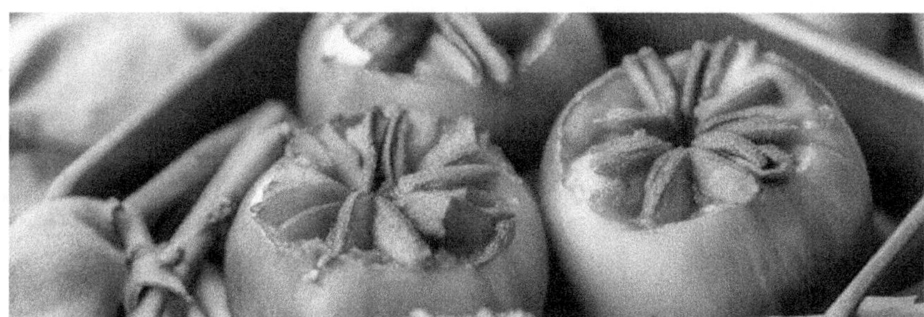

Ingredients:

- 4 large apples (such as Granny Smith or Honeycrisp)
- 2 tablespoons honey or maple syrup (adjust to taste)
- 1 teaspoon ground cinnamon
- 1/4 cup chopped nuts (such as walnuts or almonds, optional)
- Optional: a drizzle of lemon juice to prevent browning

Preparation Steps:

1. Set the oven temperature to 375°F or 190°C.

2. Give the apples a wash and core. To keep the bottoms intact, you may either use an apple core or just cut off the cores with a knife.

3. To help keep the apples' color vibrant, you may pour a little lemon juice into each one if you're worried about their browning.

4. To make a sweet and fragrant concoction, combine the ground cinnamon and honey or maple syrup in a small dish.

5. Transfer the cored apples to a baking tray and spoon the honey and cinnamon mixture into each hollow. To divide the mixture equally, you can use a spoon.

6. You may top each apple with chopped nuts if you want to add some crunch and taste.

7. Bake the baking dish in the preheated oven for 25 to 30 minutes, or until the apples are soft, covered with aluminum foil. When

they are done, they should be tender but not mushy when pierced with a fork.

8. Before serving, take the cooked apples out of the oven and let them cool somewhat.

Nutritional Values (per serving):

- Calories: About 150-200 (depending on the size of the apple)
- Sugar: About 20-25g (natural sugars from the apple and added honey or maple syrup)
- Fiber: About 4-5g
- Protein: About 1g
- Fat: About 1-2g (mostly from the nuts, if added)

Cooking Time: About 25-30 minutes

Rating: ★★★★☆ (4/5) - It's a wholesome and naturally sweet dessert!

Mixed Berry Sorbet

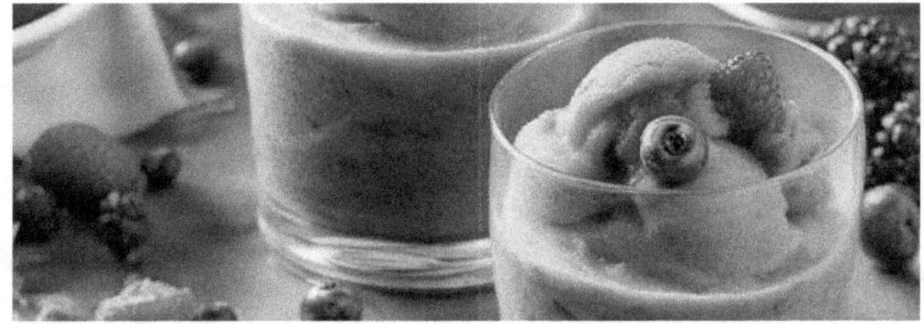

Ingredients:

- 4 large apples (such as Granny Smith or Honeycrisp)
- 2 tablespoons honey or maple syrup (adjust to taste)
- 1 teaspoon ground cinnamon
- 1/4 cup chopped nuts (such as walnuts or almonds, optional)
- Optional: a drizzle of lemon juice to prevent browning

Preparation Steps:

1. Set the oven temperature to 375°F or 190°C.
2. Give the apples a wash and core. To keep the bottoms intact, you may either use an apple core or just cut off the cores with a knife.
3. To help keep the apples' color vibrant, you may pour a little lemon juice into each one if you're worried about their browning.
4. To make a sweet and fragrant concoction, combine the ground cinnamon and honey or maple syrup in a small dish.
5. Transfer the cored apples to a baking tray and spoon the honey and cinnamon mixture into each hollow. To divide the mixture equally, you can use a spoon.
6. You may top each apple with chopped nuts if you want to add some crunch and taste.

7. Bake the baking dish in the preheated oven for 25 to 30 minutes, or until the apples are soft, covered with aluminum foil. When they are done, they should be tender but not mushy when pierced with a fork.

8. Before serving, take the cooked apples out of the oven and let them cool somewhat.

Nutritional Values (per serving):

- Calories: About 150-200 (depending on the size of the apple)
- Sugar: About 20-25g (natural sugars from the apple and added honey or maple syrup)
- Fiber: About 4-5g
- Protein: About 1g
- Fat: About 1-2g (mostly from the nuts, if added)

Cooking Time: About 25-30 minutes

Rating: ★★★★☆ (4/5) - It's a wholesome and naturally sweet dessert!

Almond and Honey Granola Bars

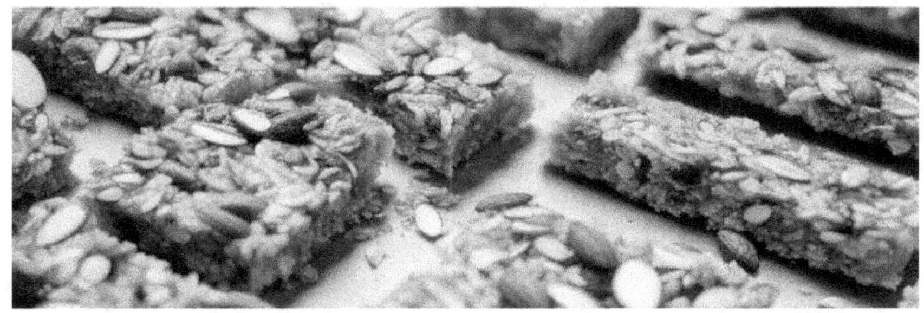

Ingredients:

- 1.5 cups rolled oats
- 1/2 cup almonds, chopped
- 1/4 cup honey
- 1/4 cup almond butter or peanut butter (unsweetened)
- 1/4 cup dried cranberries or raisins
- 1/4 cup dark chocolate chips (optional)
- 1/2 teaspoon vanilla extract
- A pinch of salt

Preparation Steps:

1. Set aside an 8x8-inch (20x20 centimeter) baking sheet and line it with parchment paper, leaving some overhang for easy removal. Preheat your oven to 350°F (175°C).

2. Place the chopped almonds and rolled oats in a large mixing dish. Arrange them equally on a baking sheet and toast for approximately 5 to 7 minutes, or until fragrant and gently brown. To avoid burning them, be careful to stir them from time to time.

3. Heat the honey and almond (or peanut) butter in a small saucepan over low heat until they are smooth and thoroughly blended. Add a little teaspoon of salt and stir in the vanilla essence.

4. Place the almonds and toasted oats, raisins or dried cranberries, and dark chocolate chips (if using) in the same large mixing bowl.

5. Top the dry ingredients in the mixing bowl with the honey and nut butter combination. Mix everything until well mixed.

6. Spoon the mixture into the ready baking pan. Firmly and evenly push it down with your hands or a spatula.

7. To give the mixture time to harden, put the pan in the fridge for a minimum of two hours.

8. After the mixture solidifies, remove the granola from the pan by using the overhanging parchment paper. After putting it on a cutting board, cut it into squares or bars.

Nutritional Values (per bar):

- Calories: About 150-200 (depending on size)
- Protein: About 3-4g
- Fat: About 7-8g (mostly from almonds and nut butter)
- Carbohydrates: About 20-25g
- Fiber: About 2-3g
- Sugar: About 10-15g (natural sugars from honey and dried fruit)

Cooking Time: About 15 minutes (plus refrigeration time)

Rating: ★★★★☆ (4/5) - It's a nutritious and satisfying snack!

Peach and Yogurt Parfait

Ingredients:

- 2 ripe peaches, peeled, pitted, and diced (or you can use canned peaches in their juice, drained)

- 1 cup Greek yogurt (unsweetened)
- 2-3 tablespoons honey or maple syrup (adjust to taste)
- 1/2 cup granola (choose a low-sugar or homemade version)
- Optional: a sprinkle of cinnamon for flavor

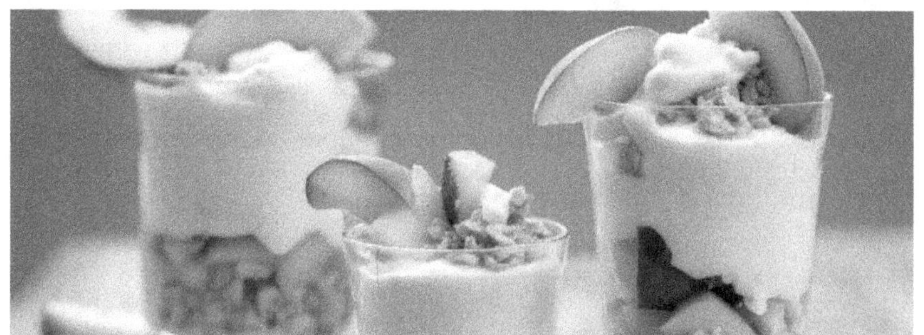

Preparation Steps:

1. Place the chopped peaches and maple syrup or honey in a bowl. Combine them to cover the peaches with the sugar. You may taste and adjust the sweetness.
2. To begin, place a tablespoon of Greek yogurt in the bottom of each serving glass or dish.
3. Cover the yogurt with a layer of the chopped peaches that have been sweetened.
4. Cover the peaches with a layer of granola. This provides a nice crunch and texture.
5. Repeat the layers until you fill the glass or bowl, concluding with a final dollop of Greek yogurt on top.

6. If you want to add even more taste, you may optionally sprinkle some cinnamon on top.

7. To enable the flavors to mingle together, chill the parfaits in the fridge for at least half an hour before serving.

Nutritional Values (per serving):

- Calories: About 250-300 (depending on serving size and granola)
- Protein: About 10g
- Fat: About 5-6g (mostly from yogurt and granola)
- Carbohydrates: About 45-50g
- Fiber: About 3-4g
- Sugar: About 30-35g (natural sugars from peaches and added sweetener)

Preparation Time: About 10-15 minutes (plus chilling time)

Rating: ★★★★★ (5/5) - It's a creamy and fruity delight!

Dark Chocolate-Dipped Strawberries

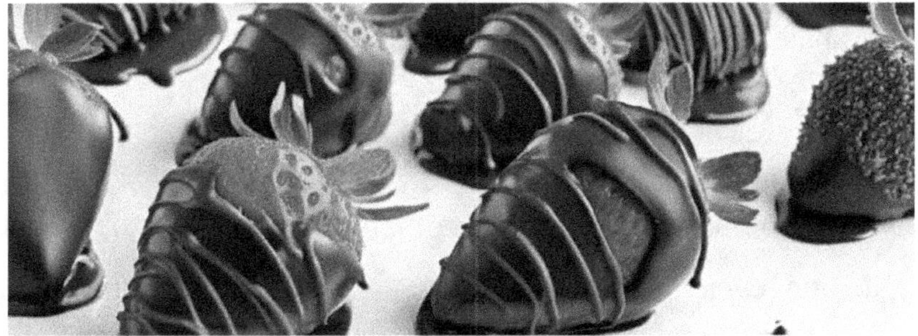

Ingredients:

- 12-16 fresh strawberries, washed and dried (leave the stems on for easy dipping)
- 4 ounces (about 113 grams) of dark chocolate (70% cocoa or higher)
- Optional: white chocolate or chopped nuts for drizzling or rolling (adjust to taste)

Preparation Steps:

1. Use wax or parchment paper to line a baking sheet or tray. This is where the dipped strawberries will be placed to cool.

2. In a microwave-safe basin or using a double boiler, melt the dark chocolate. When heating chocolate in a microwave, do it in 20–30 second bursts, stirring in between, until the chocolate is melted and smooth.

3. Holding each strawberry by its stem, immerse it into the melted chocolate, spinning to cover it evenly. Let any dripping chocolate fall back into the bowl.

4. Transfer each dipped strawberry to the baking sheet or pan that has been ready.

5. You may dip the strawberries in dark chocolate and then roll them in chopped nuts while the chocolate is still soft if you want to add even more flare. You can also drizzle melted white chocolate over the strawberries.

6. Let the strawberries that have been dipped cool and solidify. To expedite the procedure, you may put them in the refrigerator for around thirty minutes.

Nutritional Values (per strawberry, with dark chocolate):

- Calories: About 50-60
- Sugar: About 4-5g
- Fat: About 3-4g (mostly from the chocolate)
- Carbohydrates: About 7-8g
- Fiber: About 1-2g
- Protein: About 1g

Cooking Time: About 15-20 minutes (including cooling time)

Rating: ★★★★★ (5/5) - It's a decadent and elegant dessert!

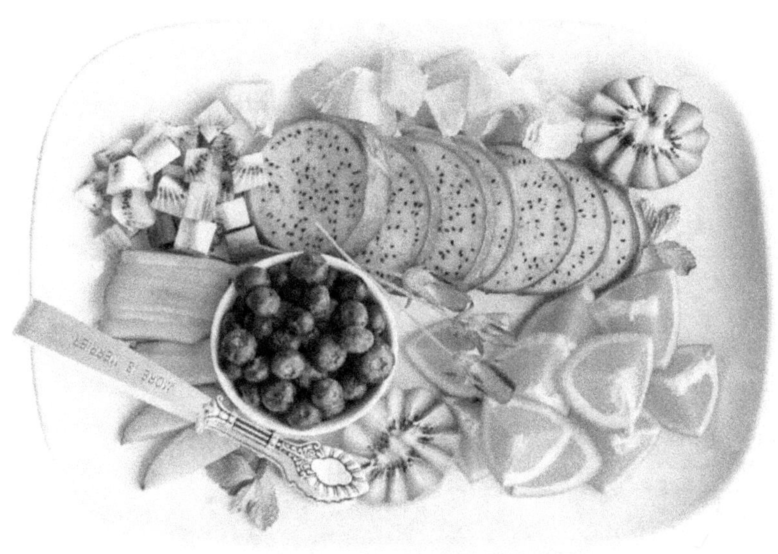

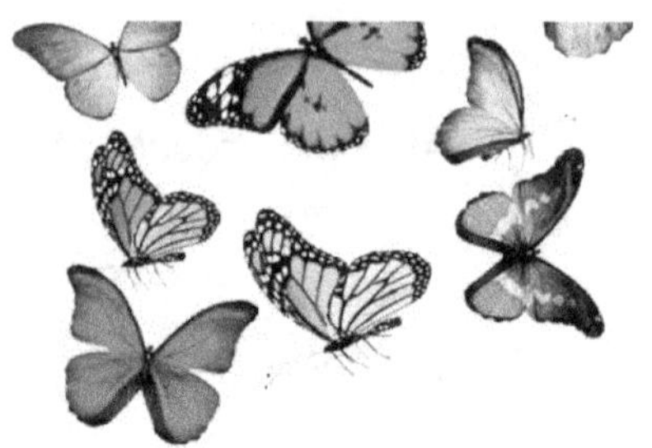

"Facing gout head-on with dietary changes shows incredible resilience. Remember, you're making choices that benefit not just your joints, but your overall health. Embrace the variety and richness of anti-inflammatory foods. Every healthy choice is a positive step towards healing. It's a journey of discovery – of new flavors, habits, and a healthier you. Stay patient, stay consistent, and trust the process. You're on the right path!"

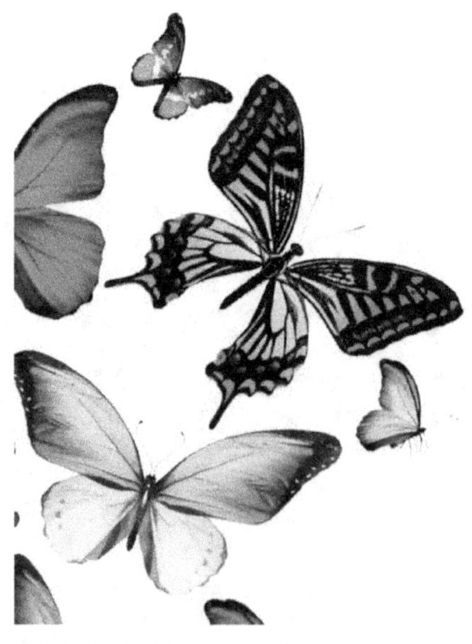

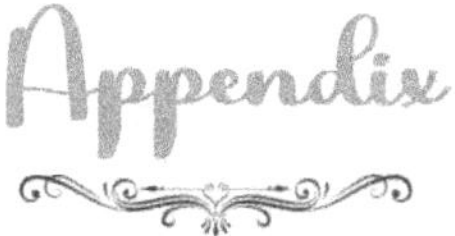

Appendix

28-Days Meal Planning and Prep for Gout Management

This plan includes a variety of meals to keep your taste buds satisfied while following a gout-conscious diet.

Day 1:

- **Breakfast:** Cherry-Banana Oatmeal

- **Lunch:** Tofu Stir-Fry with Brown Rice

- **Dinner:** Turkey Meatballs with Zucchini Noodles

- **Snack:** Roasted Mixed Nuts

- **Dessert:** Dark Chocolate-Dipped Strawberries

Day 2:

- **Breakfast:** Spinach and Feta Whole Wheat Wraps

- **Lunch:** Whole Wheat Turkey Sandwich with Cucumber and Sprouts

- **Dinner:** Tomato and Basil Sauce on Whole Wheat Pasta

- **Snack:** Cucumber and Chickpea Salad

- **Dessert:** Peach and Yogurt Parfait

Day 3:

- **Breakfast:** Scrambled Eggs with Avocado on Toast

- **Lunch:** Lentil and Vegetable Soup

- **Dinner:** Vegetable and Bean Chili

- **Snack:** Baked Sweet Potato Fries

- **Dessert:** Almond and Honey Granola Bars

Day 4:

- **Breakfast:** Whole Grain Blueberry Pancakes

- **Lunch:** Grilled Chicken and Mixed Greens Salad

- **Dinner:** Baked Chicken Breast with Quinoa and Asparagus

- **Snack:** Fresh Fruit Salad

- **Dessert:** Mixed Berry Sorbet

Day 5:

- **Breakfast:** Greek Yogurt with Mixed Berries and Nuts

- **Lunch:** Quinoa and Roasted Vegetable Salad

- **Dinner:** Grilled Salmon with Steamed Broccoli

- **Snack:** Carrot and Celery Sticks with Hummus

- **Dessert:** Baked Apples with Cinnamon

- (Continue this pattern, rotating through the meal options for breakfast, lunch, dinner, snacks, and desserts, ensuring each day offers a different combination.)

Day 6 to Day 28:

- Follow a similar rotation, ensuring each meal category (breakfast, lunch, dinner, snack, dessert) has a different option each day. After using all options in a category, start again from the first option.

For example:

Day 6:

- **Breakfast:** Cherry-Banana Oatmeal

- **Lunch:** Tofu Stir-Fry with Brown Rice

- **Dinner:** Tomato and Basil Sauce on Whole Wheat Pasta

- **Snack:** Roasted Mixed Nuts

- **Dessert:** Dark Chocolate-Dipped Strawberries

Day 7:

- **Breakfast:** Spinach and Feta Whole Wheat Wraps

- **Lunch:** Whole Wheat Turkey Sandwich with Cucumber and Sprouts

- **Dinner:** Vegetable and Bean Chili

- **Snack:** Cucumber and Chickpea Salad

- **Dessert:** Peach and Yogurt Parfait

(Continue this pattern for days 8-28.)

General Notes:

- From Day 15 onwards, introduce new dinner options like Teriyaki Glazed Salmon, Seafood Paella, and Lean Beef Fajitas for variety.

- Rotate the snack and dessert options so you're not having the same item two days in a row.

- Remember to adjust portion sizes and ingredients according to personal dietary needs and preferences.

- Stay hydrated and consult with a healthcare provider for any specific dietary requirements related to gout management.

This plan provides a varied and balanced diet suitable for managing gout, incorporating a wide range of nutrients and flavors while maintaining a focus on low-purine foods.

Understanding and Managing Uric Acid Levels

Consider uric acid to be your body's natural waste product. It develops as a result of your body breaking down specific compounds known as purines, which are created by your body and present in some diets.

Uric acid has two purposes. It has anti-oxidant properties that are beneficial to your health. However, too much of it might be problematic, particularly if you have gout.

Linking Gout and Uric Acid:

Gout is a kind of arthritis that develops when crystals of uric acid lodge in your joints. These crystals have the potential to be problematic since they hurt and irritate. Blood uric acid levels over normal raise the likelihood of developing gout.

Controlling Acidity Levels:

Let's now discuss ways to control those uric acid levels:

1. Pay Attention to Your Diet:

Reduce your intake of purine-rich foods such as organ meats, red meat, shellfish, and certain vegetables like spinach and asparagus.

Instead, aim for healthful grains, fruits, vegetables, and dairy products.

2. Monitor Your Body Weight:

If you must drop weight, do it gradually and with medical assistance if necessary.

3. Use Sugary Drinks and Alcohol Caution:

It's advisable to minimize or avoid beer as it might induce gout.

Additionally, reduce your intake of fructose-containing foods and beverages since these may raise your uric acid levels.

4. Drugs:

Sometimes, your doctor could prescribe medicines to assist manage uric acid. There are several types, such as those that aid in your kidneys' removal of uric acid or ones that reduce its creation.

You may need to use NSAIDs or colchicine to relieve discomfort if your gout flares up.

5. Well-Being Lifestyle:

Regular exercise can help you stay in shape and lower your chance of developing gout.

Learn stress management techniques since these can prevent gout episodes.

6. Pay Attention to Your Levels:

Periodically, your doctor will want to check your uric acid levels to evaluate how things are progressing.

7. Drink Plenty of Water:

Getting adequate water into your body aids in the removal of uric acid.

8. Tailored Method:

Recall that managing your gout is specific to you. Together with your healthcare practitioner, develop a strategy that is tailored to your need.

9. No Sudden Diets:

Avoid such crash diets; they can actually bring on gout episodes. The best approach is to lose weight steadily and gradually.

Thus, you may control your gout and lead a more pleasant and healthy life by controlling your uric acid levels. Remember to keep your doctor updated; they are there to support you all the way!

Supplements and Natural Remedies

When it comes to gout, there are several supplements and natural therapies that may help alleviate symptoms and lessen the frequency of gout episodes. Consider the following:

1. Cherry Extract:

Cherries, whether consumed whole or as cherry extract supplements, have been related to decreased uric acid levels and a lower incidence of gout episodes.

You can eat fresh cherries or consult your doctor about cherry extract supplements.

2. Vitamin C:

Some people's uric acid levels can be reduced by taking vitamin C. You may obtain your daily dosage from citrus fruits, strawberries, or supplements if your doctor recommends it.

3. Fish oil (Omega-3 Fatty Acids):

Omega-3 fatty acids, present in fish oil supplements, offer anti-inflammatory characteristics that may aid with gout-related inflammation.

Before incorporating fish oil supplements into your daily regimen, check with your doctor.

4. Turmeric:

Curcumin, the main ingredient in turmeric, has anti-inflammatory qualities and may give relief from gout symptoms.

After consulting with your healthcare professional, you can add turmeric to your meals or consider curcumin pills.

5. Devil's Claw:

Devil's claw is a traditional herbal treatment recognized for its anti-inflammatory properties. Some folks find it beneficial for gout.

Before attempting herbal therapies, always speak with your healthcare physician.

6. Stinging Nettle:

Another herbal medicine that has been used to treat gout symptoms is stinging nettle. It may assist to lessen inflammation.

Before using stinging nettle, see your doctor.

7. Bromelain:

Bromelain, an enzyme present in pineapple, may have anti-inflammatory qualities and may be useful to gout sufferers.

Consult your doctor before using bromelain pills.

8. Hydration and Diet:

Staying hydrated and maintaining a gout-friendly diet, as previously noted, are natural therapies in and of themselves. They can help avoid gout attacks.

Remember:

- While these supplements and natural therapies may provide comfort to some people, their efficacy varies from person to person.

- It is critical to contact with your healthcare professional before beginning any new supplements or cures, especially if you have underlying health concerns or are using drugs.

- Gout management should be thorough and personalized to your unique needs, so always collaborate with your healthcare team to develop the best strategy for you.

- Incorporating these vitamins and natural therapies, with the supervision of your healthcare professional, can be a complimentary strategy to controlling gout and improving your overall well-being.

Lifestyle Changes and Exercise for Gout Prevention

Gout is a type of arthritis that can be managed and even prevented through some key lifestyle changes. Here's what you can do:

1. **Diet Modification:**

   - **Limit Purine-Rich Foods:** Foods high in purines, like red meat, organ meats, shellfish, and certain vegetables, can raise uric acid levels. Reducing these in your diet is a smart move.

- **Embrace Low-Purine Foods:** On the flip side, focus on low-purine foods like whole grains, fruits, vegetables, and dairy products.

- **Moderate Alcohol:** Alcohol, especially beer, can trigger gout attacks. If you choose to drink, do so in moderation.

2. Hydration:

- Staying well-hydrated is vital. Water helps your body flush out excess uric acid. Aim for at least 8-10 glasses of water daily.

3. Weight Management:

- Maintaining a healthy weight is essential. Excess weight can contribute to higher uric acid levels and increase your risk of gout. Gradual, steady weight loss can be beneficial.

4. Sugar and Fructose:

- Cut back on sugary drinks and foods high in fructose, as they can raise uric acid levels.

5. Medications:

- If you've had gout attacks before, your doctor might prescribe medications to lower uric acid levels or prevent flares.

Exercise for Gout Prevention:

Regular exercise is a powerful tool in the fight against gout. Here's how it helps:

1. **Weight Control:**

    - Exercise helps you maintain a healthy weight or lose excess pounds, reducing your risk of gout.

2. **Improved Joint Function:**

    - Physical activity keeps your joints moving, improving their function and reducing the risk of gout-related joint damage.

3. **Lower Inflammation:**

    - Exercise can help lower overall inflammation in your body, which is beneficial for gout management.

4. **Enhanced Insulin Sensitivity:**

    - Some studies suggest that exercise can improve insulin sensitivity, potentially reducing uric acid levels.

5. **Cardiovascular Health:**

    - Gout is often associated with other health issues like heart disease and diabetes. Regular exercise supports overall cardiovascular health, reducing these risks.

Types of Exercise for Gout:

Here are some exercise options to consider:

1. **Low-Impact Aerobics:**

   - Activities like walking, swimming, and cycling are easy on the joints while providing cardiovascular benefits.

2. **Strength Training:**

   - Building muscle through weightlifting or resistance exercises can improve joint stability and overall strength.

3. **Flexibility Exercises:**

   - Gentle stretching and yoga can help maintain joint flexibility and reduce stiffness.

4. **Stay Active Daily:**

   - Incorporate movement into your daily life. Take the stairs, go for short walks, or do some light household chores.

5. **Listen to Your Body:**

   - Be mindful of your body's signals. If you experience joint pain during or after exercise, adjust your routine and consult your doctor.

Remember:

- Always consult with your healthcare provider before starting a new exercise program, especially if you have existing health conditions or concerns about gout.

- Start gradually and build up your exercise routine to avoid overexertion and minimize the risk of gout flares.

By making these lifestyle changes and incorporating regular exercise, you can significantly reduce your risk of gout attacks and enjoy improved overall health. It's all about finding a balance that works for you and your unique needs.

For further Questions and advice reach out on
joanmilonehelpdesk@gmail.com

Thank You

I'm writing this with a heart full of gratitude for your kind words and the time you took to read my book, knowing that my words have resonated with you is a reward beyond measure. Thank you again for your appreciation and for being a part of this literary journey.

Warmly,

Joan

30 Days
Meal
Planner

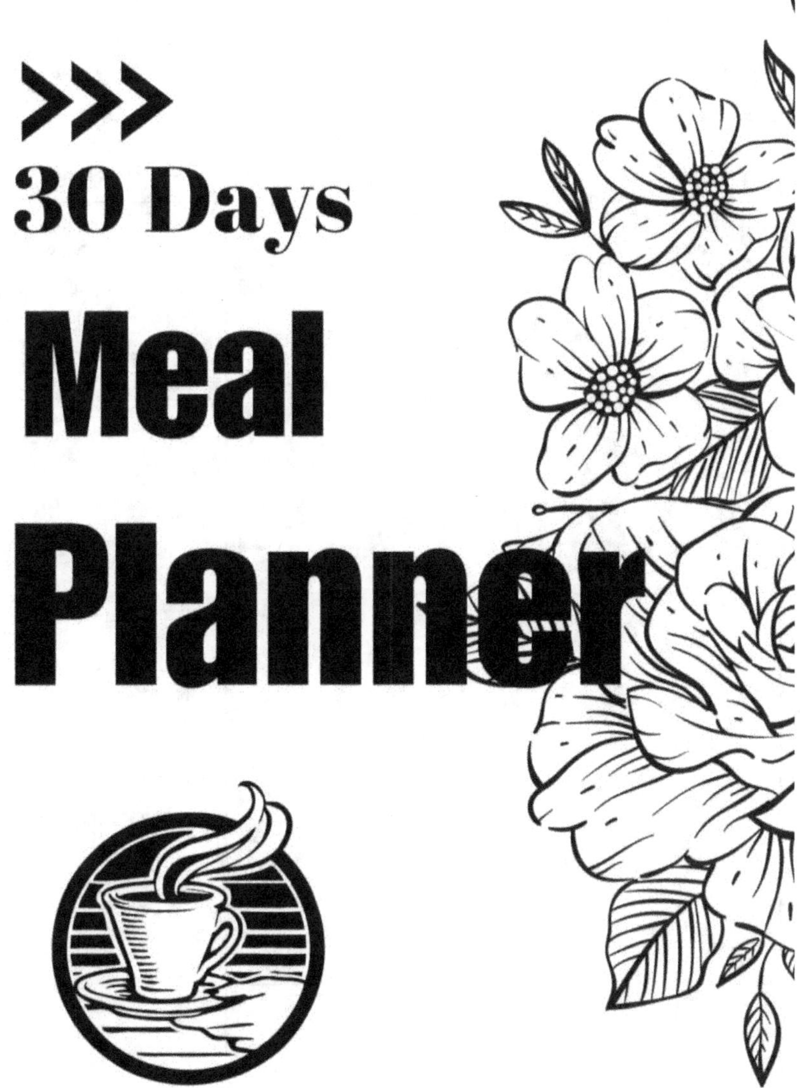

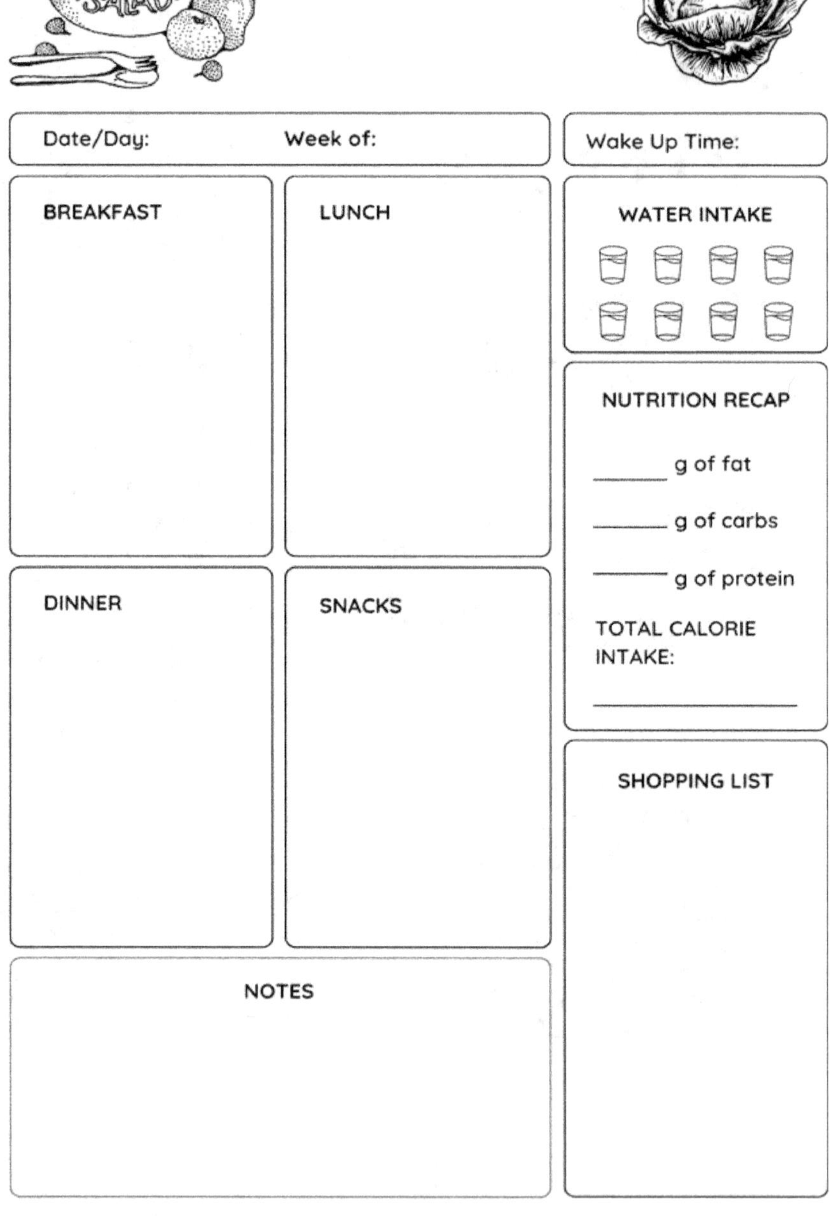

| Date/Day: | Week of: | Wake Up Time: |

BREAKFAST

LUNCH

WATER INTAKE

NUTRITION RECAP

_________ g of fat

_________ g of carbs

_________ g of protein

TOTAL CALORIE INTAKE:

____

DINNER

SNACKS

SHOPPING LIST

NOTES

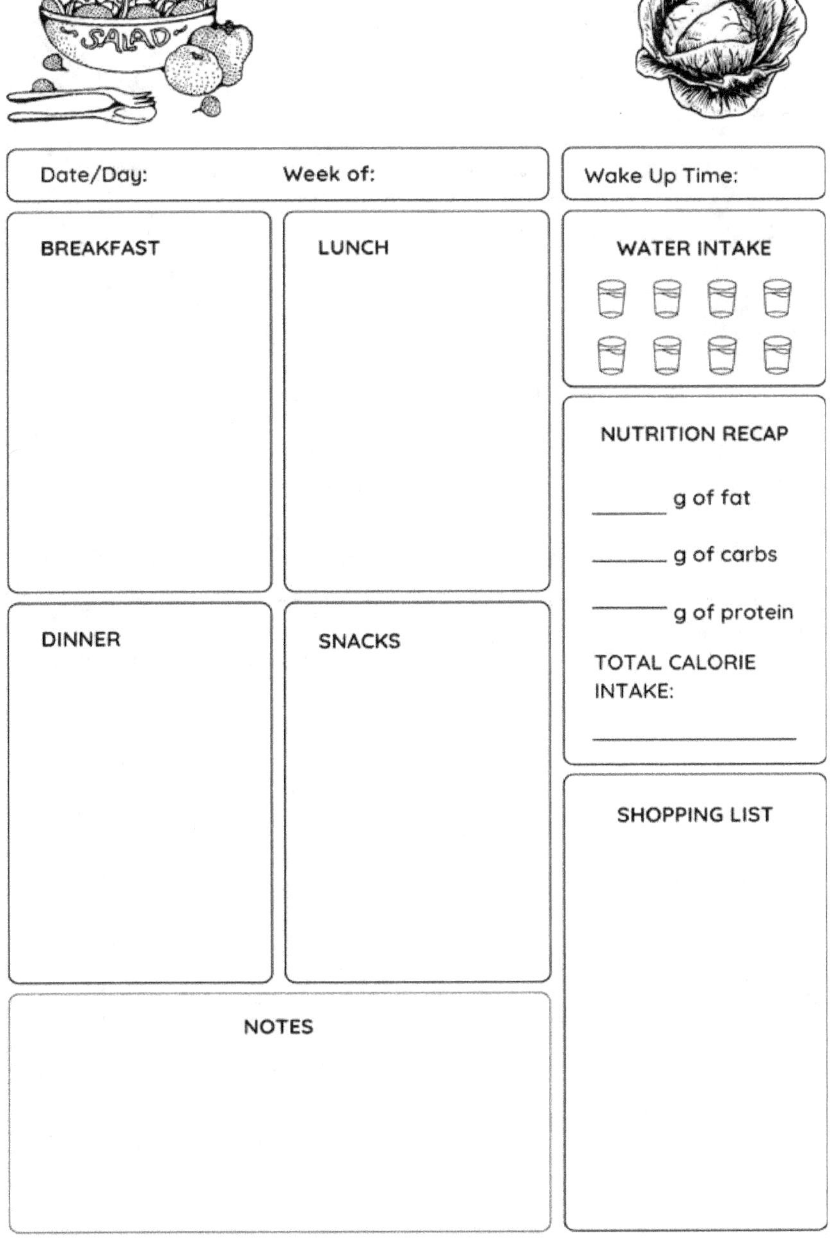

| Date/Day: | Week of: | Wake Up Time: |

BREAKFAST

LUNCH

WATER INTAKE

NUTRITION RECAP

_______ g of fat

_______ g of carbs

_______ g of protein

TOTAL CALORIE INTAKE:

DINNER

SNACKS

SHOPPING LIST

NOTES

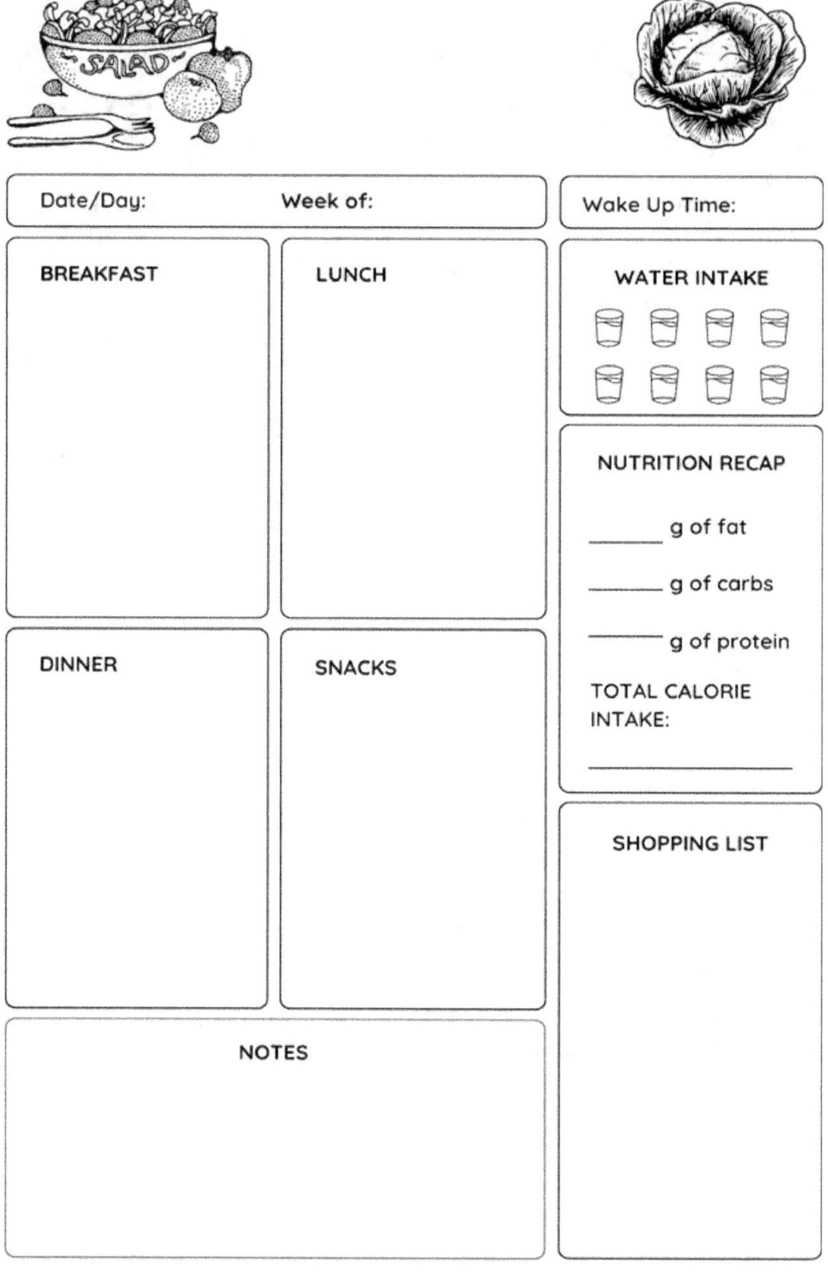

| Date/Day: | Week of: | Wake Up Time: |

BREAKFAST

LUNCH

WATER INTAKE

NUTRITION RECAP

_______ g of fat

_______ g of carbs

_______ g of protein

TOTAL CALORIE INTAKE:

DINNER

SNACKS

SHOPPING LIST

NOTES

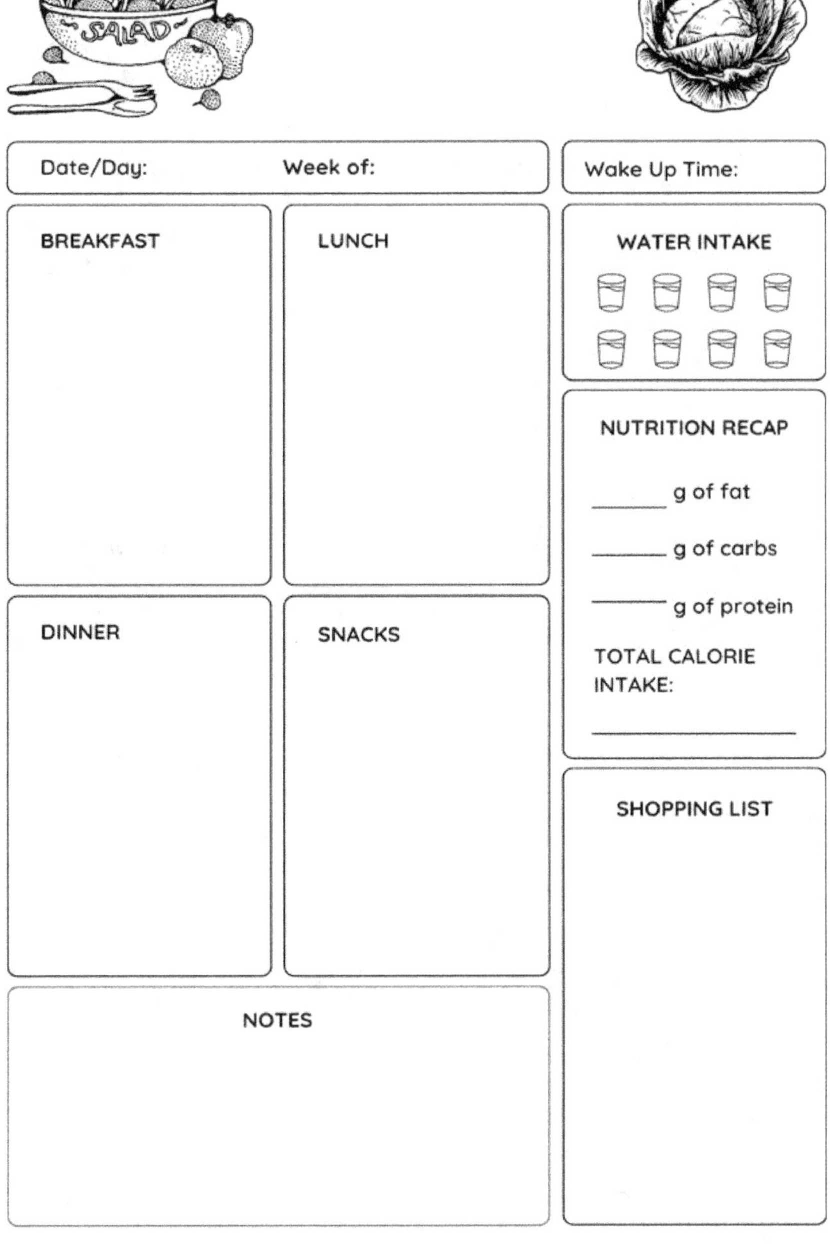

| Date/Day: | Week of: | Wake Up Time: |

BREAKFAST

LUNCH

WATER INTAKE

NUTRITION RECAP

______ g of fat

______ g of carbs

______ g of protein

TOTAL CALORIE INTAKE:

____

DINNER

SNACKS

SHOPPING LIST

NOTES

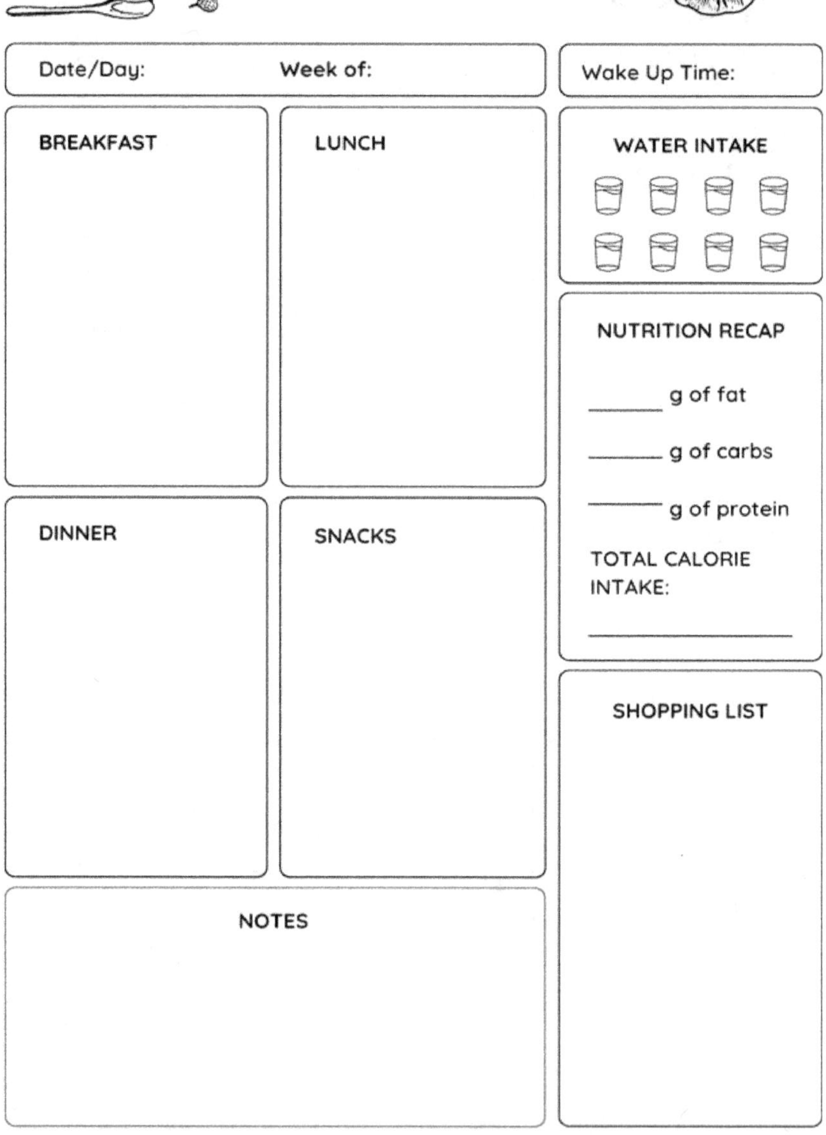

| Date/Day: | Week of: | Wake Up Time: |

BREAKFAST

LUNCH

WATER INTAKE

NUTRITION RECAP

_______ g of fat

_______ g of carbs

_______ g of protein

TOTAL CALORIE INTAKE:

____

DINNER

SNACKS

SHOPPING LIST

NOTES

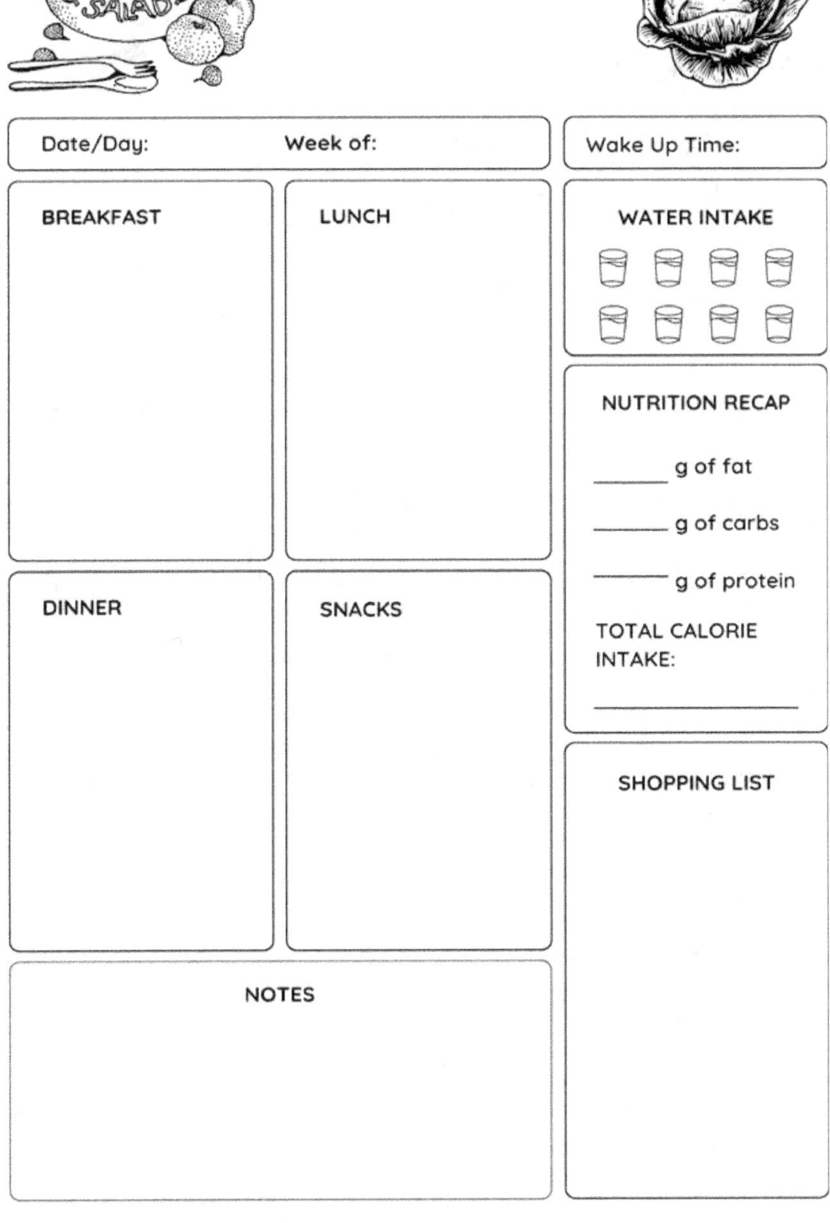

Date/Day: Week of:
Wake Up Time:
BREAKFAST
LUNCH
WATER INTAKE
NUTRITION RECAP
_______ g of fat
_______ g of carbs
_______ g of protein
TOTAL CALORIE INTAKE:
DINNER
SNACKS
SHOPPING LIST
NOTES

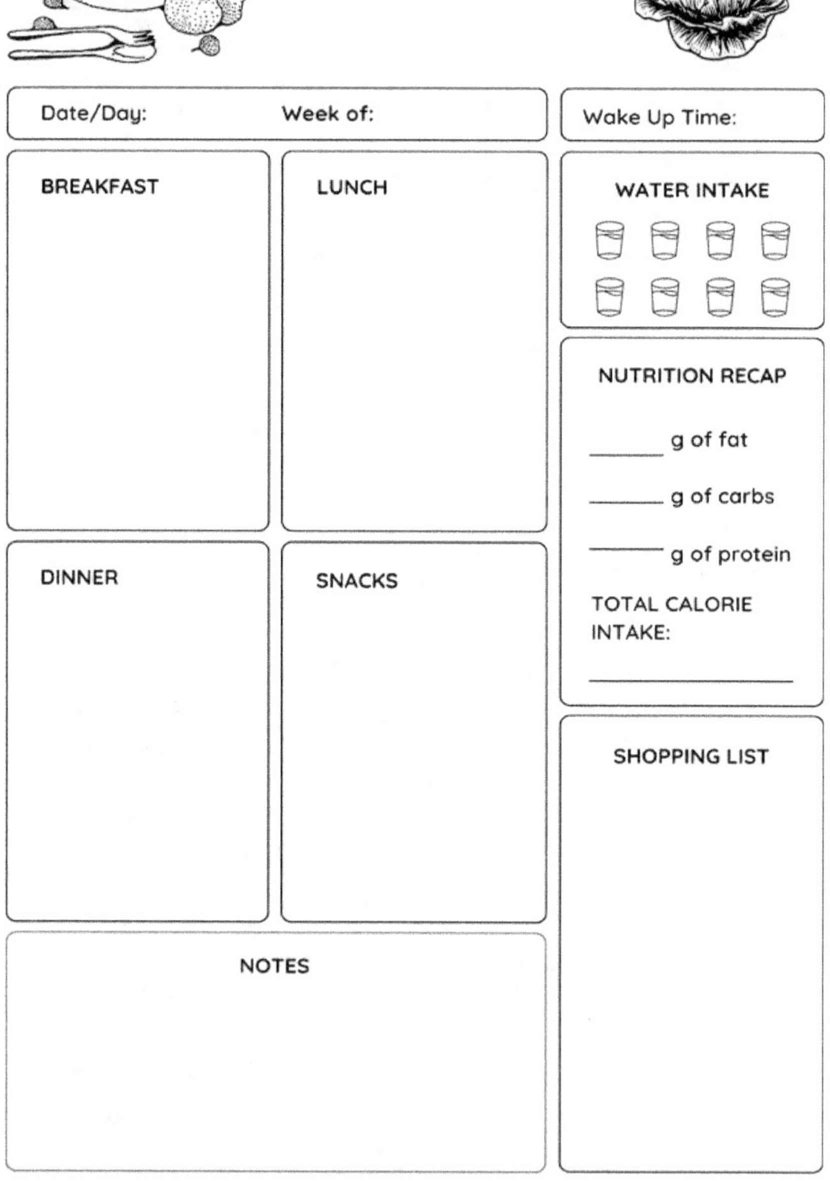

| Date/Day: | Week of: | Wake Up Time: |

BREAKFAST

LUNCH

WATER INTAKE

NUTRITION RECAP

_______ g of fat

_______ g of carbs

_______ g of protein

TOTAL CALORIE INTAKE:

____

DINNER

SNACKS

SHOPPING LIST

NOTES

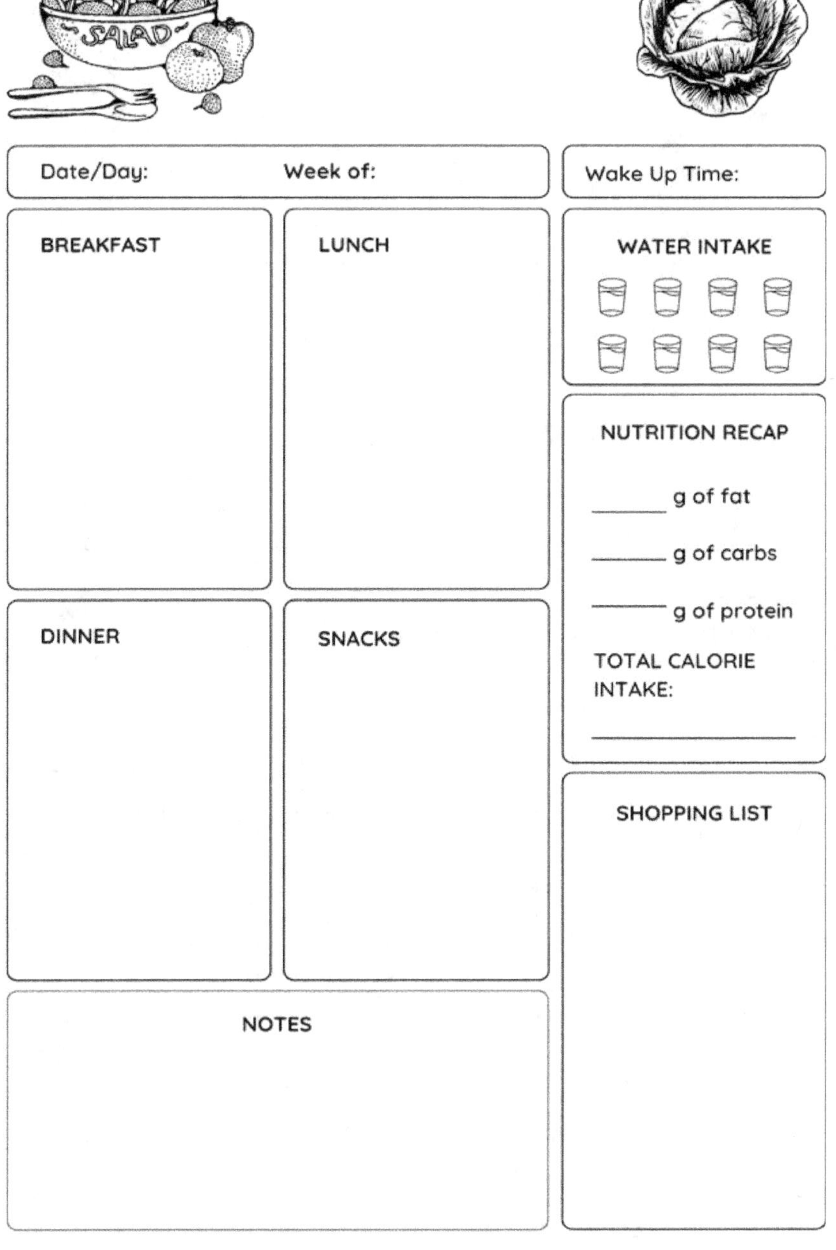

Date/Day:
Week of:
Wake Up Time:
BREAKFAST
LUNCH
WATER INTAKE
NUTRITION RECAP
_______ g of fat
_______ g of carbs
_______ g of protein
TOTAL CALORIE INTAKE:
DINNER
SNACKS
SHOPPING LIST
NOTES

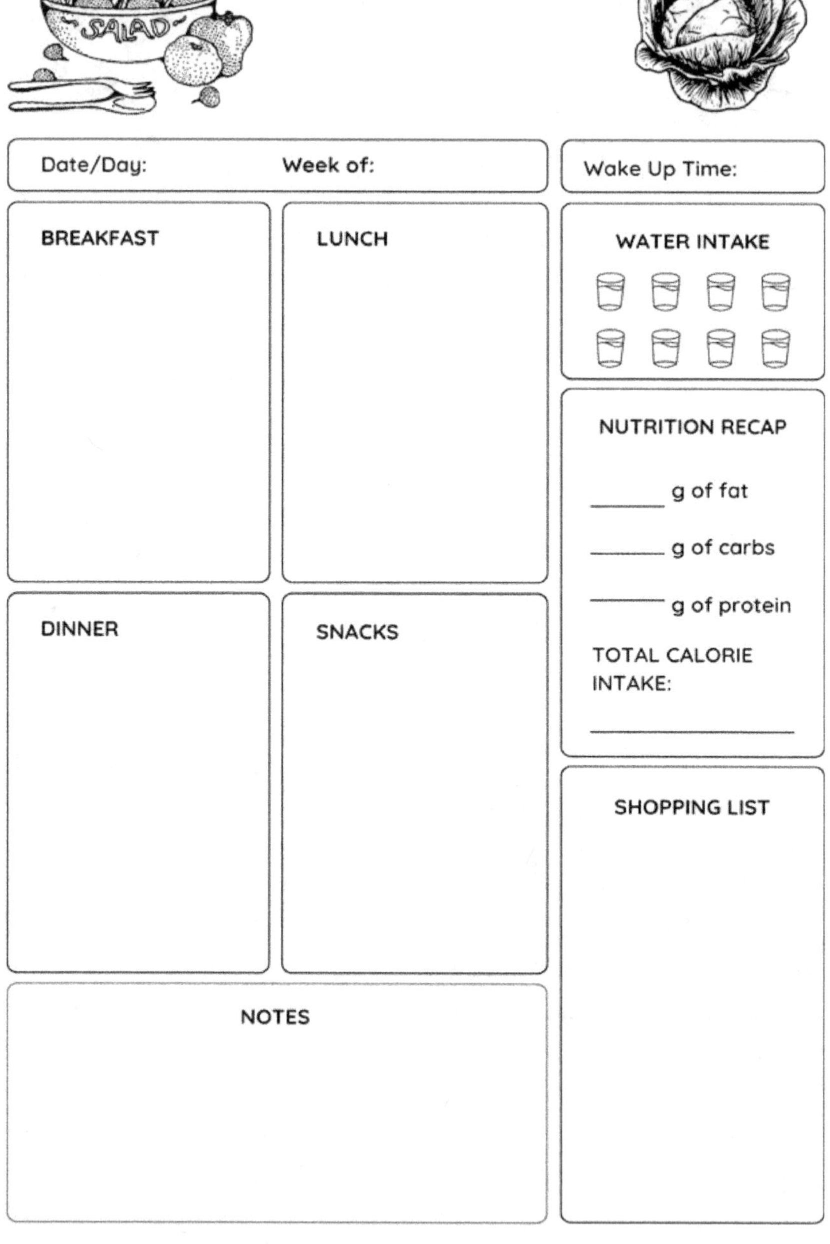
SALAD
Date/Day:
Week of:
Wake Up Time:
BREAKFAST
LUNCH
WATER INTAKE
NUTRITION RECAP
_______ g of fat
_______ g of carbs
_______ g of protein
TOTAL CALORIE INTAKE:
DINNER
SNACKS
SHOPPING LIST
NOTES

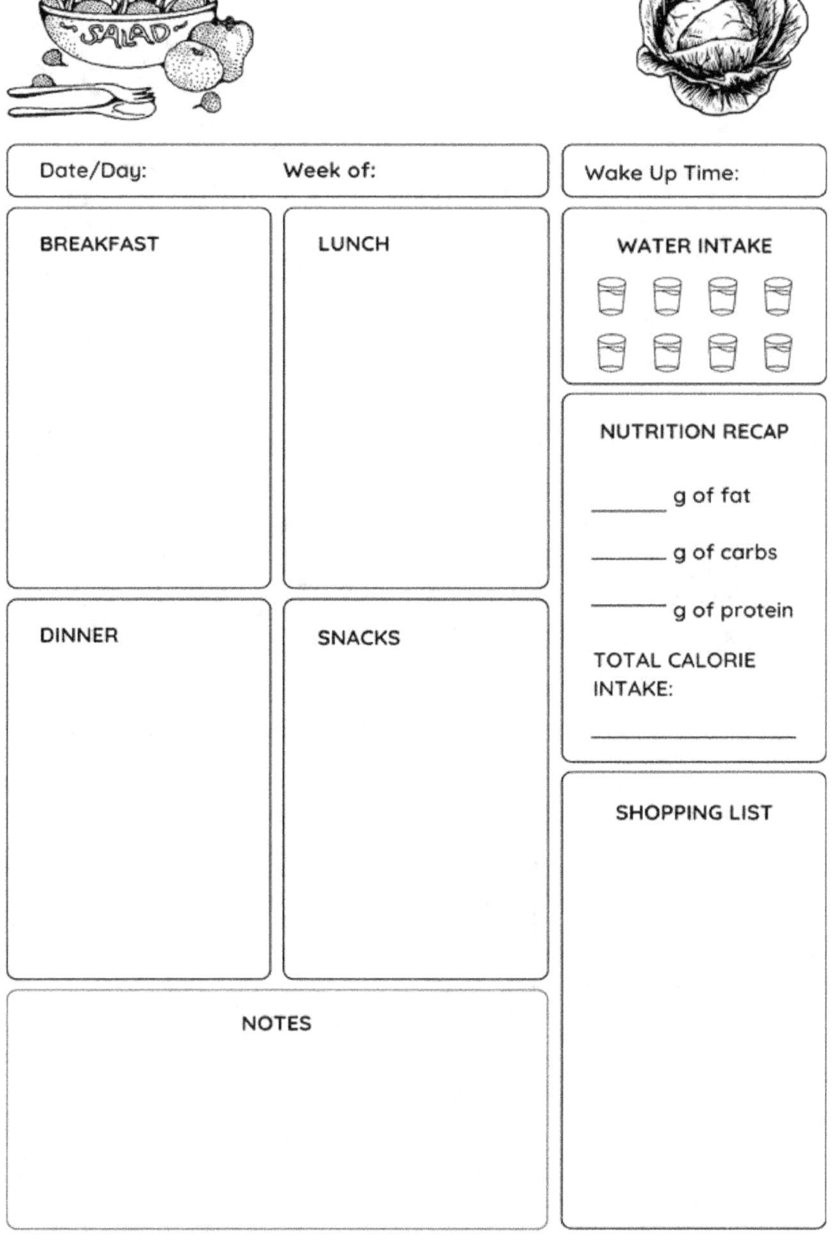

| Date/Day: | Week of: | Wake Up Time: |

BREAKFAST

LUNCH

WATER INTAKE

NUTRITION RECAP

_______ g of fat

_______ g of carbs

_______ g of protein

TOTAL CALORIE INTAKE:

____

DINNER

SNACKS

SHOPPING LIST

NOTES

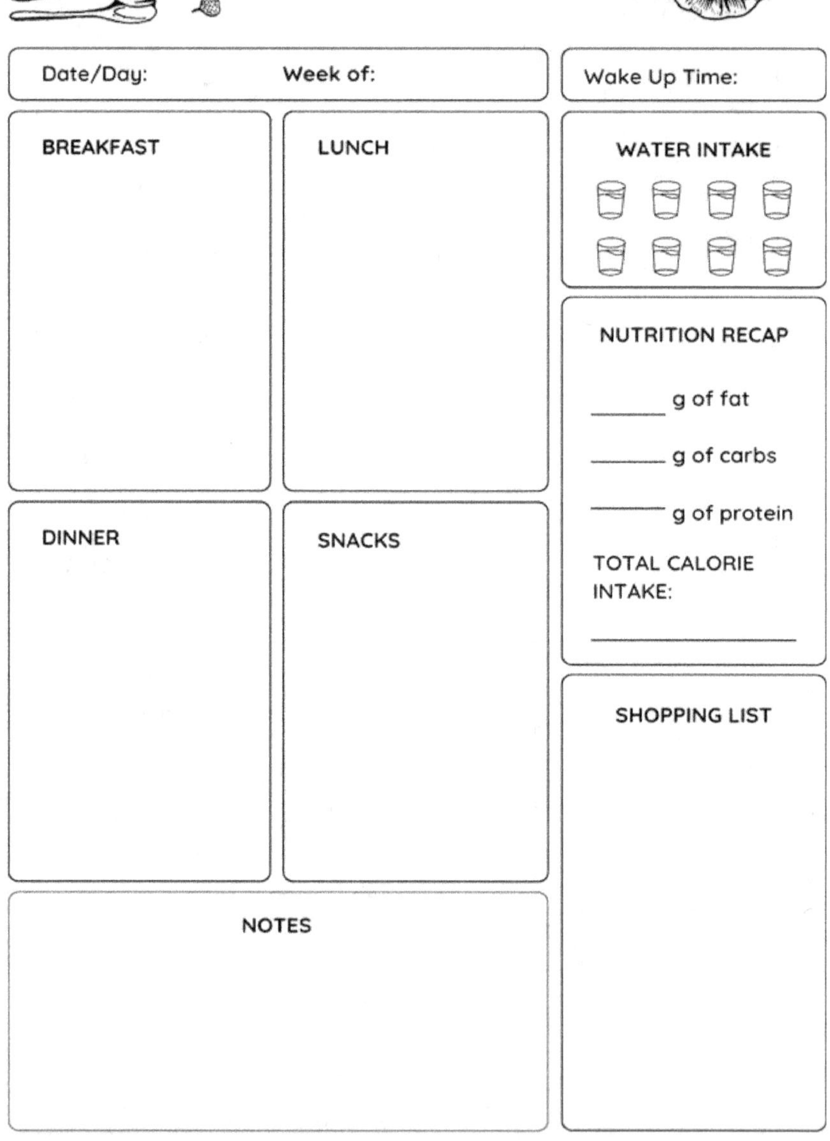

| Date/Day: | Week of: | Wake Up Time: |

BREAKFAST

LUNCH

WATER INTAKE

DINNER

SNACKS

NUTRITION RECAP

_______ g of fat

_______ g of carbs

_______ g of protein

TOTAL CALORIE INTAKE:

____

SHOPPING LIST

NOTES

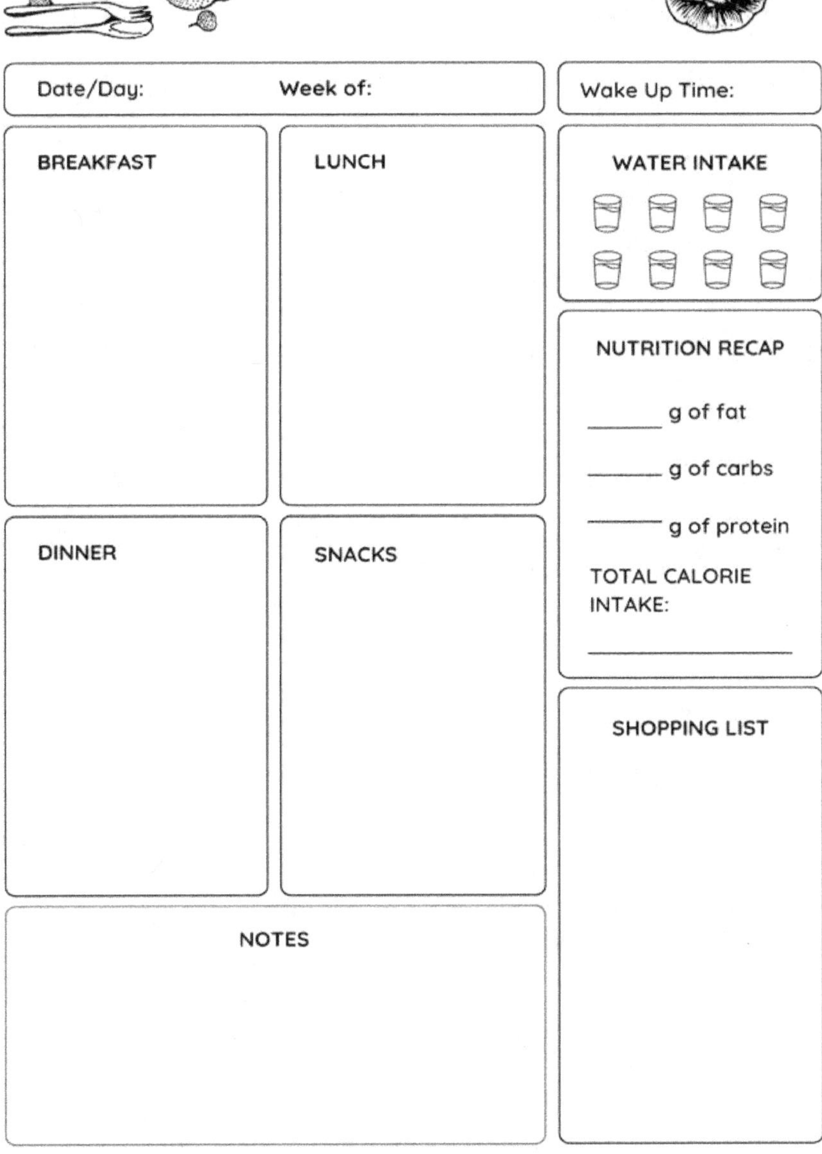

Date/Day:
Week of:
Wake Up Time:
BREAKFAST
LUNCH
WATER INTAKE
NUTRITION RECAP
________ g of fat
________ g of carbs
________ g of protein
TOTAL CALORIE INTAKE:
DINNER
SNACKS
SHOPPING LIST
NOTES

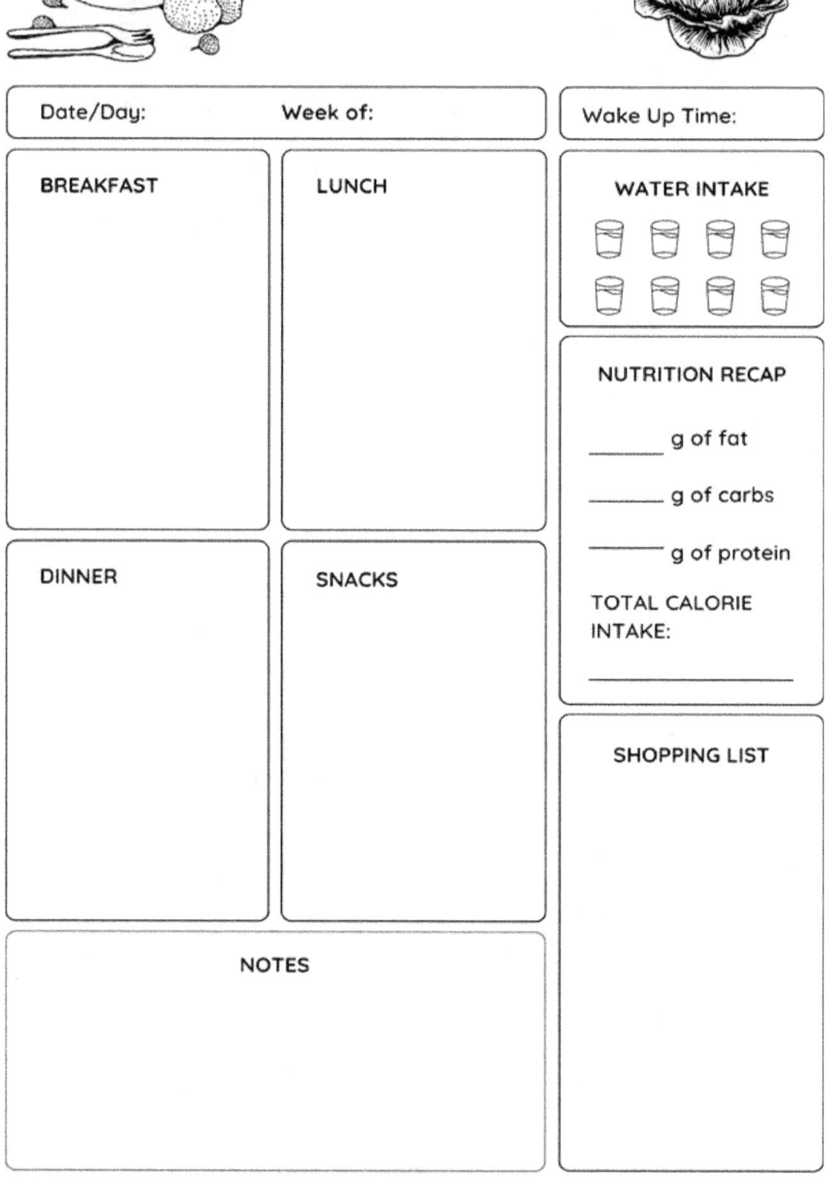

Date/Day: Week of:

Wake Up Time:

BREAKFAST

LUNCH

WATER INTAKE

NUTRITION RECAP

______ g of fat

______ g of carbs

______ g of protein

TOTAL CALORIE INTAKE:

____

DINNER

SNACKS

SHOPPING LIST

NOTES

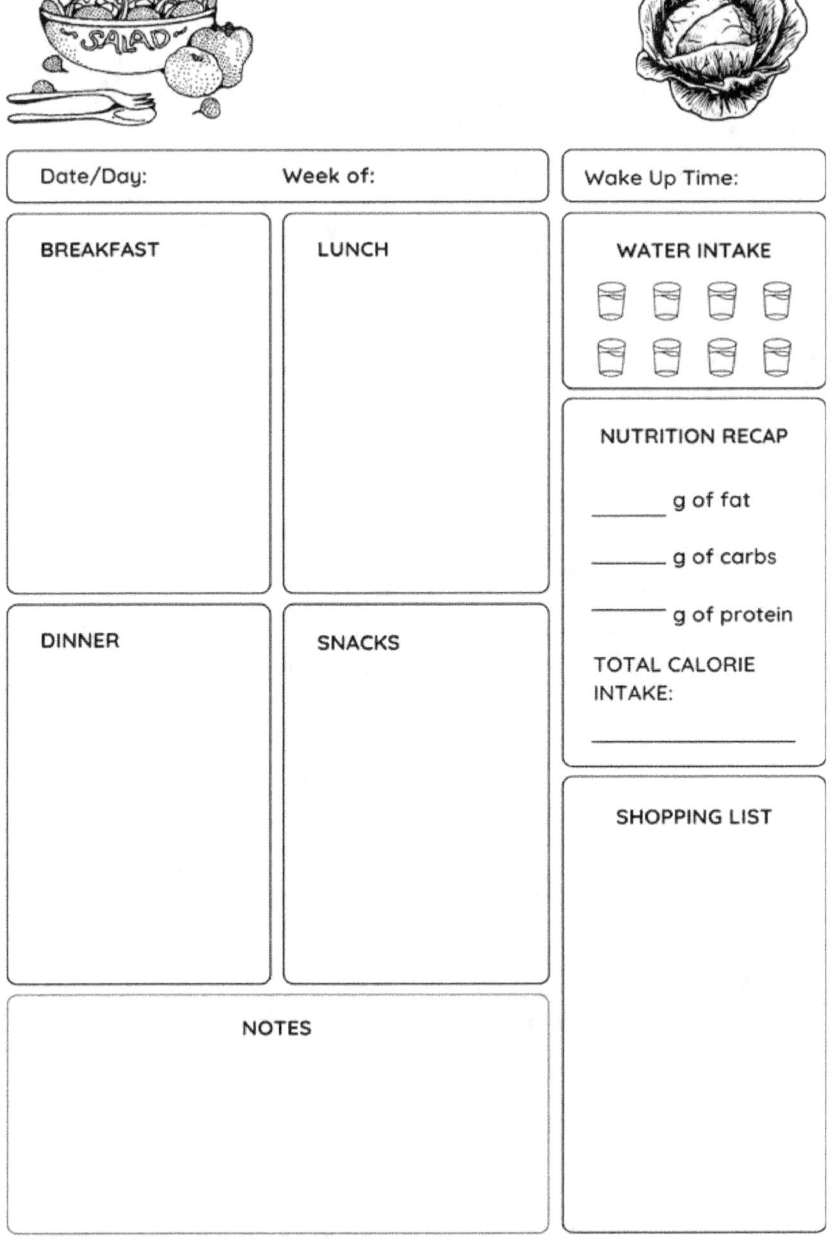

| Date/Day: | Week of: | Wake Up Time: |

BREAKFAST

LUNCH

WATER INTAKE

NUTRITION RECAP

______ g of fat

______ g of carbs

______ g of protein

TOTAL CALORIE INTAKE:

____

DINNER

SNACKS

SHOPPING LIST

NOTES

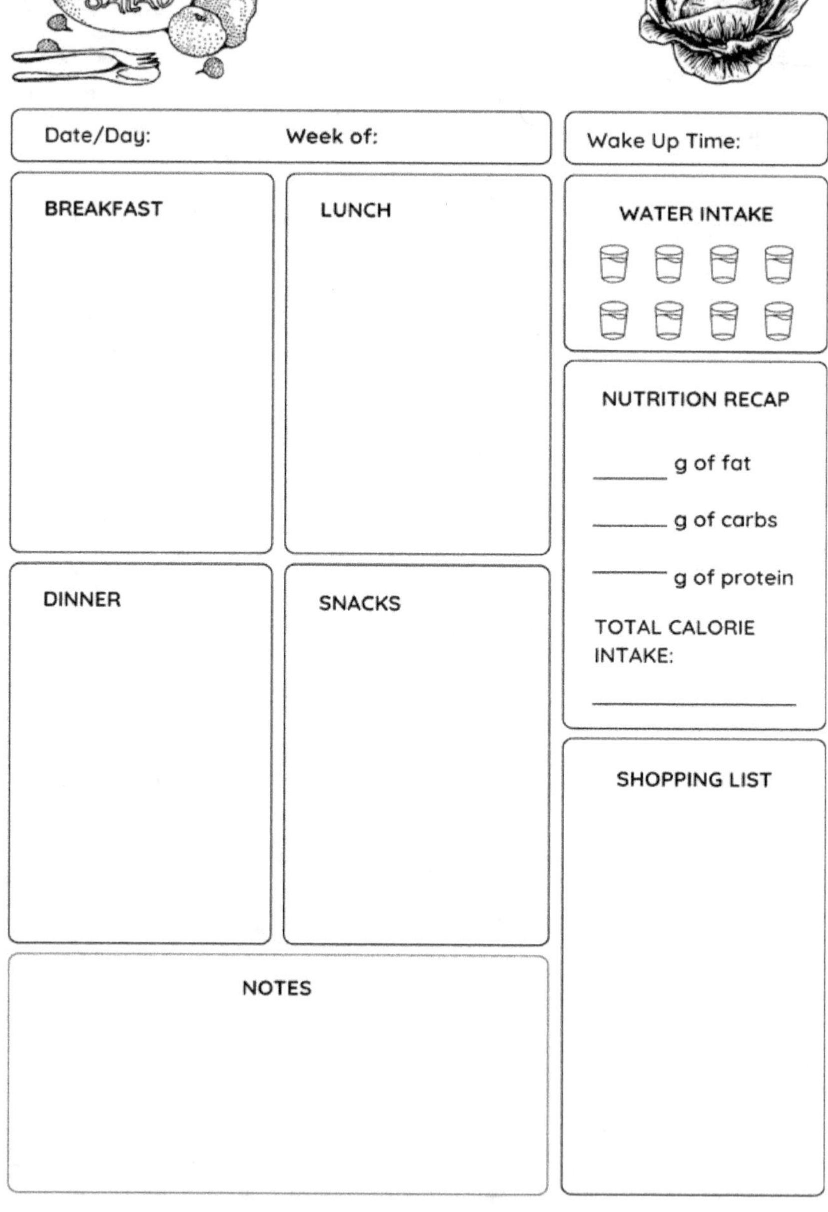

Date/Day:
Week of:
Wake Up Time:
BREAKFAST
LUNCH
WATER INTAKE
DINNER
SNACKS
NUTRITION RECAP
_______ g of fat
_______ g of carbs
_______ g of protein
TOTAL CALORIE INTAKE:
____
SHOPPING LIST
NOTES

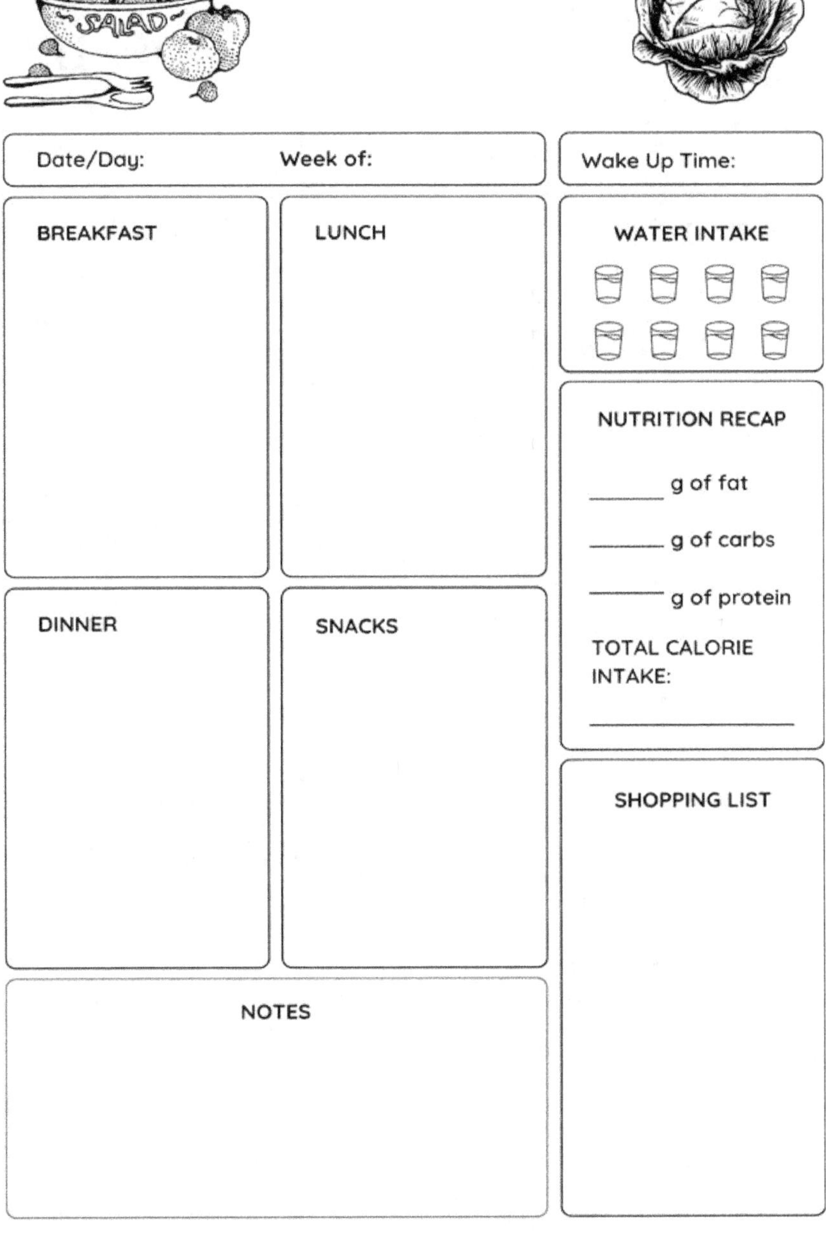
Date/Day:
Week of:
Wake Up Time:
BREAKFAST
LUNCH
WATER INTAKE
NUTRITION RECAP
_______ g of fat
_______ g of carbs
_______ g of protein
TOTAL CALORIE INTAKE:
DINNER
SNACKS
SHOPPING LIST
NOTES

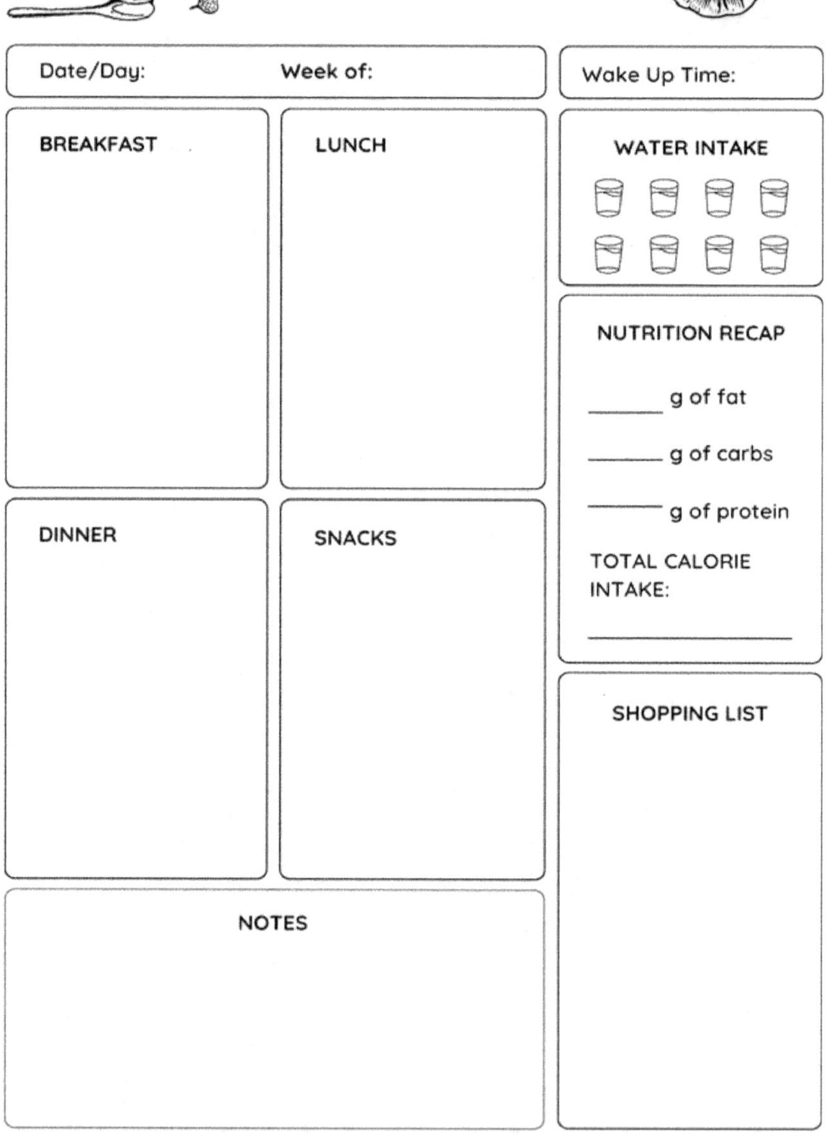

| Date/Day: | Week of: | Wake Up Time: |

BREAKFAST

LUNCH

WATER INTAKE

NUTRITION RECAP

_______ g of fat

_______ g of carbs

_______ g of protein

TOTAL CALORIE INTAKE:

DINNER

SNACKS

SHOPPING LIST

NOTES

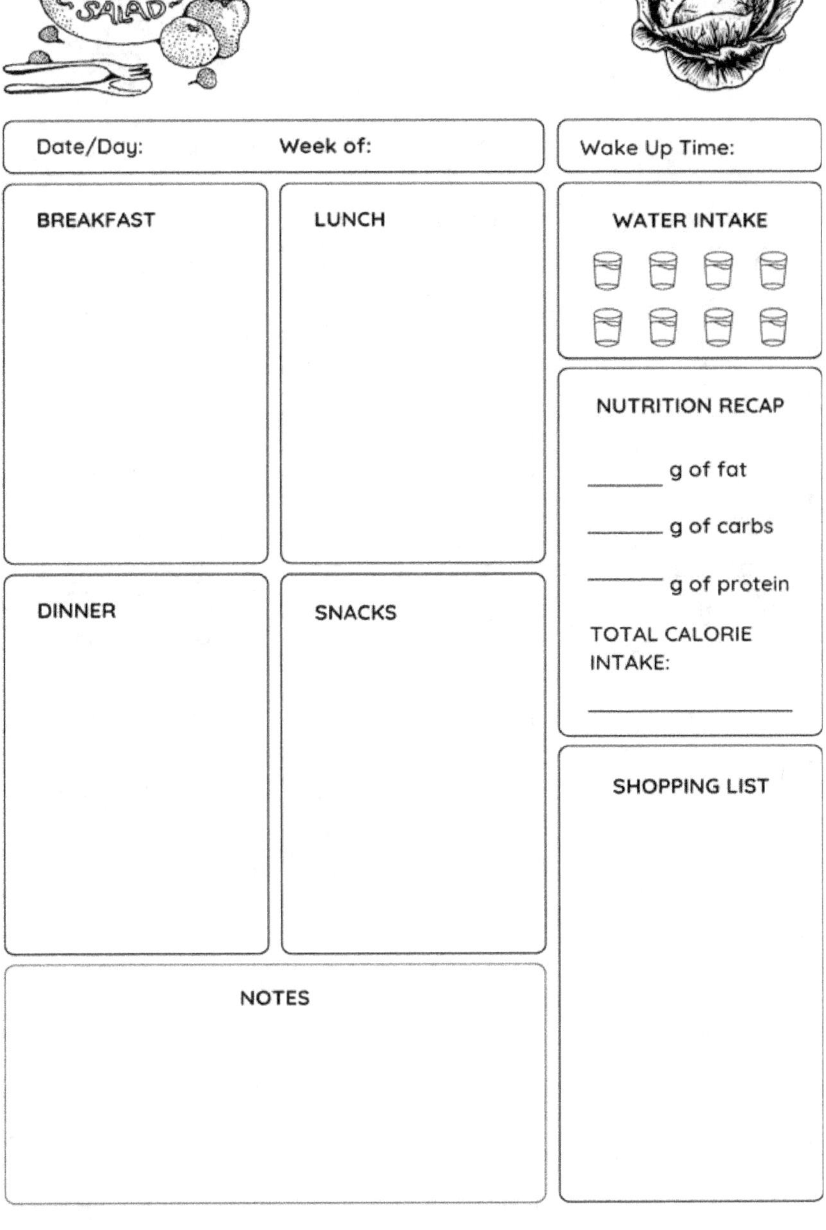

| Date/Day: | Week of: | Wake Up Time: |

BREAKFAST

LUNCH

WATER INTAKE

NUTRITION RECAP

_______ g of fat

_______ g of carbs

_______ g of protein

TOTAL CALORIE INTAKE:

____

DINNER

SNACKS

SHOPPING LIST

NOTES

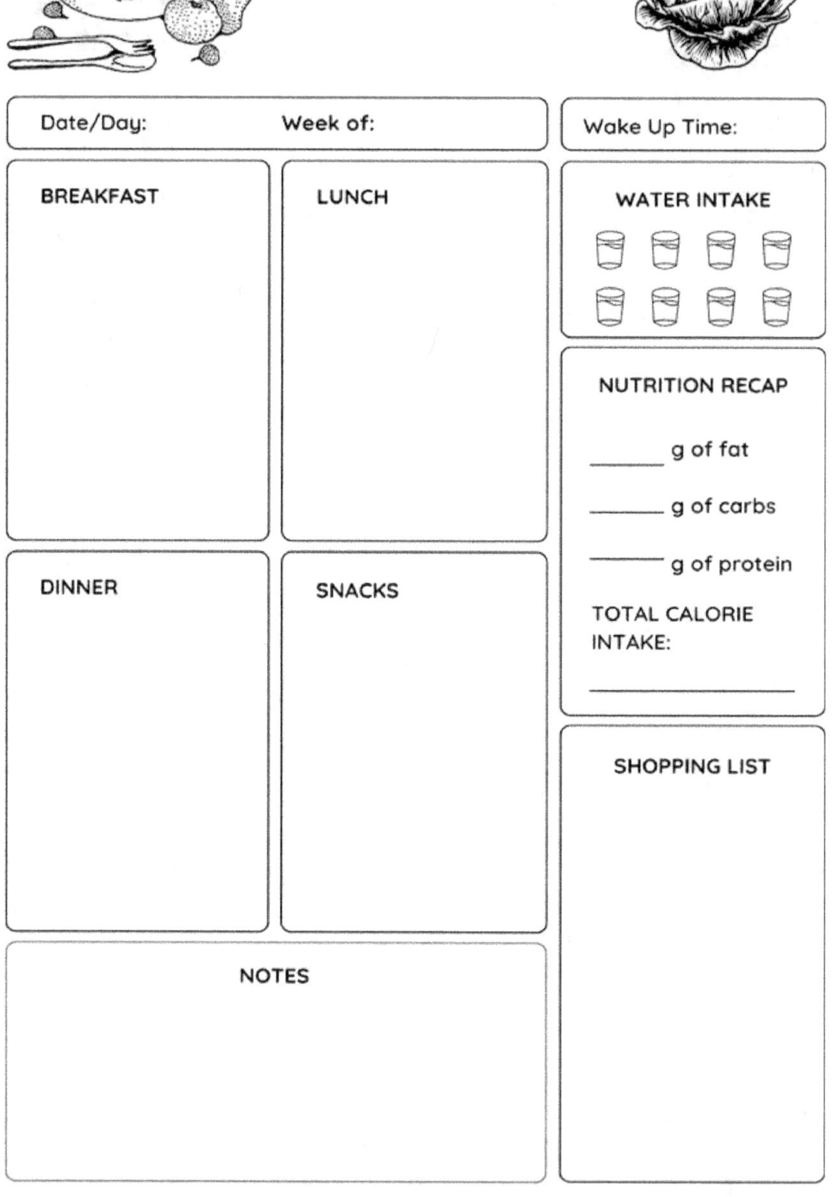

Date/Day:	Week of:

Wake Up Time:

BREAKFAST

LUNCH

WATER INTAKE

NUTRITION RECAP

______ g of fat

______ g of carbs

______ g of protein

TOTAL CALORIE INTAKE:

____

DINNER

SNACKS

SHOPPING LIST

NOTES

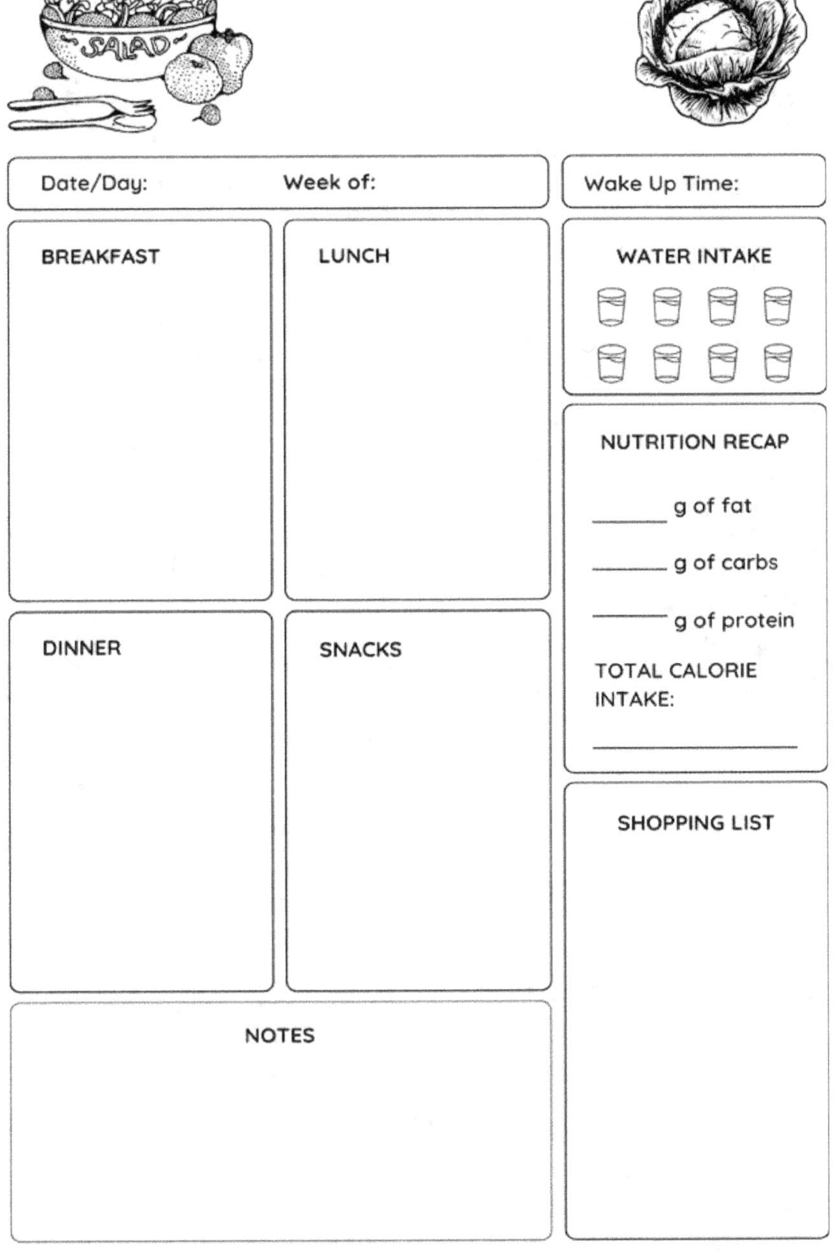

| Date/Day: | Week of: | Wake Up Time: |

BREAKFAST

LUNCH

WATER INTAKE

NUTRITION RECAP

________ g of fat

________ g of carbs

________ g of protein

TOTAL CALORIE INTAKE:

____

DINNER

SNACKS

SHOPPING LIST

NOTES

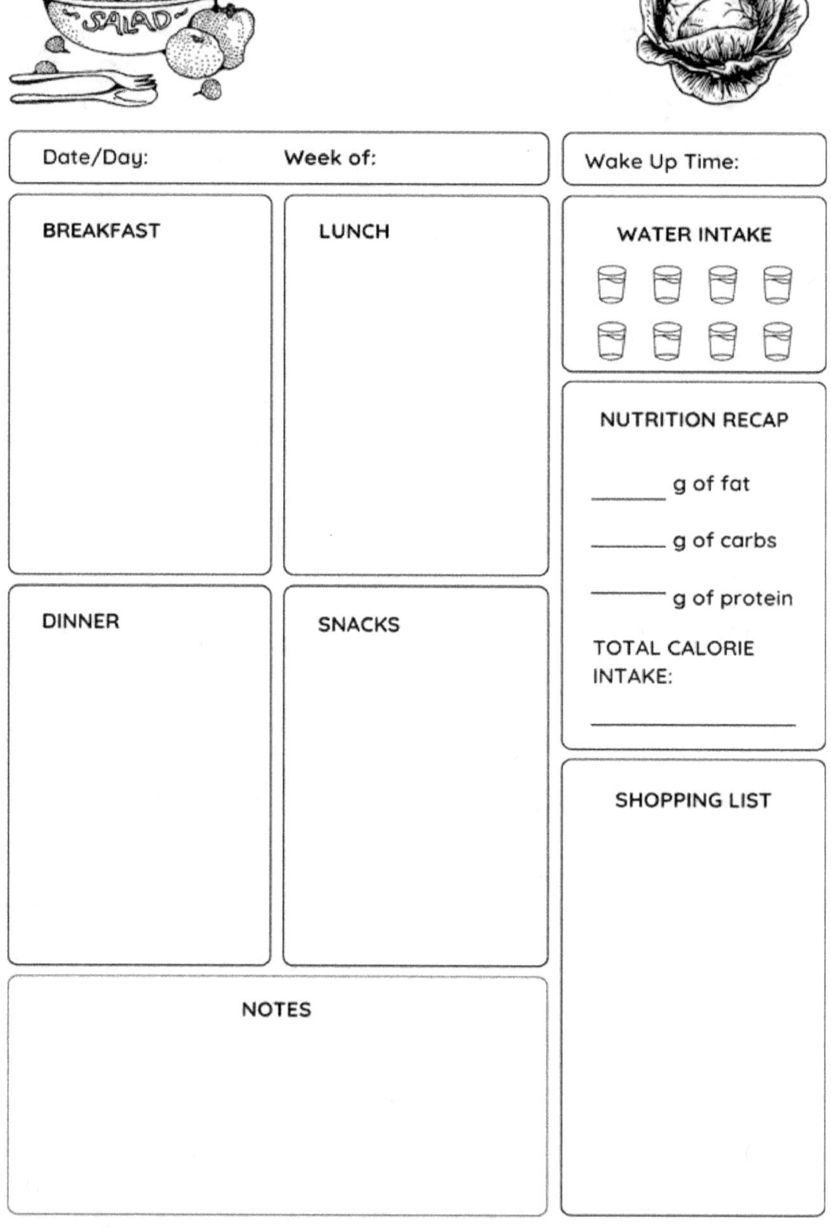

Date/Day: Week of:

Wake Up Time:

BREAKFAST

LUNCH

WATER INTAKE

NUTRITION RECAP

__________ g of fat

__________ g of carbs

__________ g of protein

TOTAL CALORIE INTAKE:

DINNER

SNACKS

SHOPPING LIST

NOTES

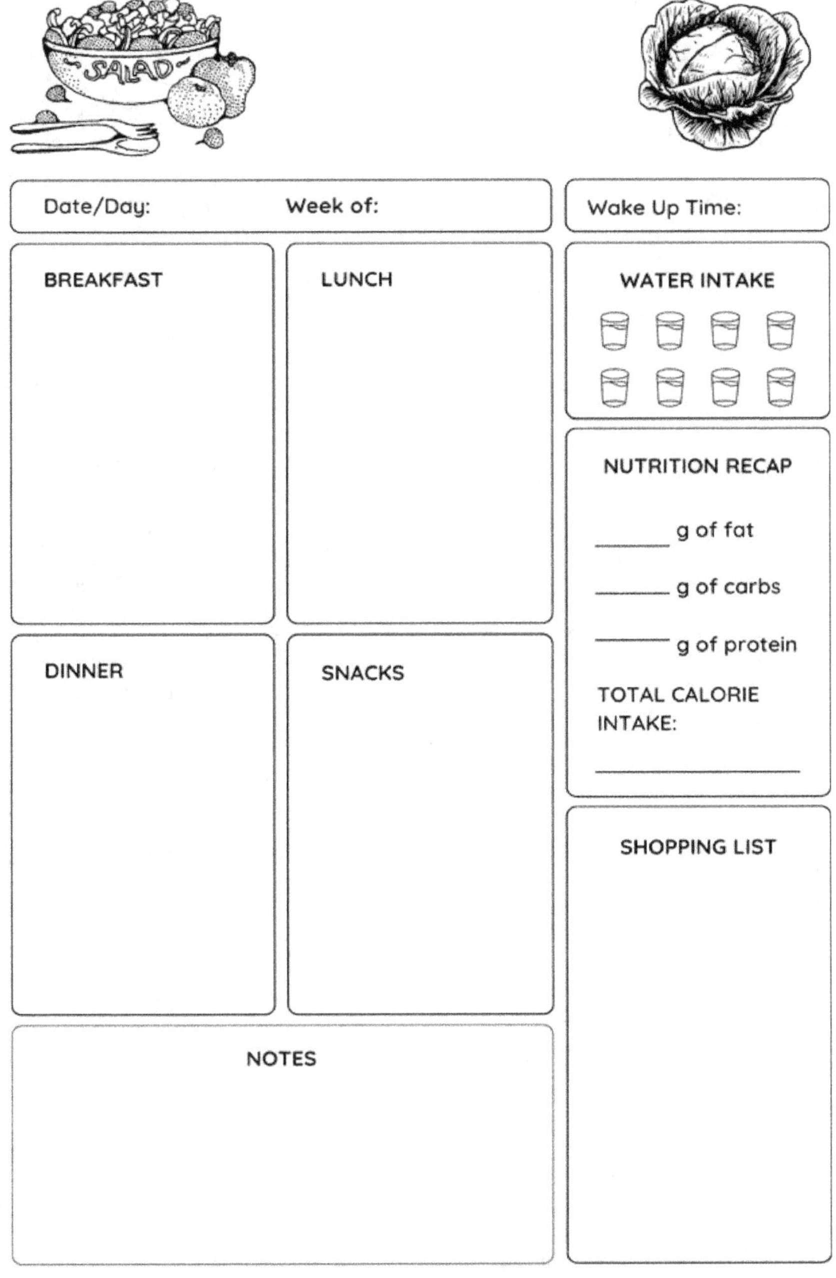

Date/Day:	Week of:

Wake Up Time:

BREAKFAST

LUNCH

WATER INTAKE

NUTRITION RECAP

_________ g of fat

_________ g of carbs

_________ g of protein

TOTAL CALORIE INTAKE:

____

DINNER

SNACKS

SHOPPING LIST

NOTES

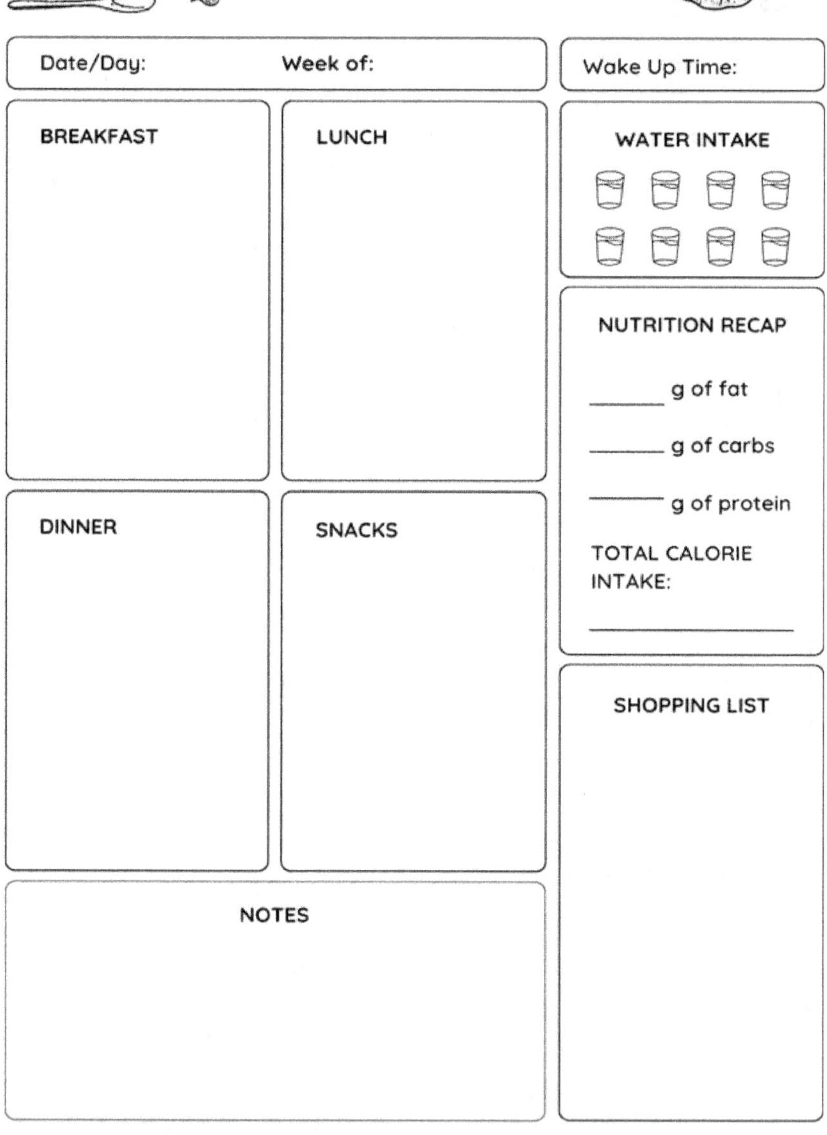

| Date/Day: | Week of: | Wake Up Time: |

BREAKFAST

LUNCH

WATER INTAKE

NUTRITION RECAP

______ g of fat

______ g of carbs

______ g of protein

TOTAL CALORIE INTAKE:

____

DINNER

SNACKS

SHOPPING LIST

NOTES

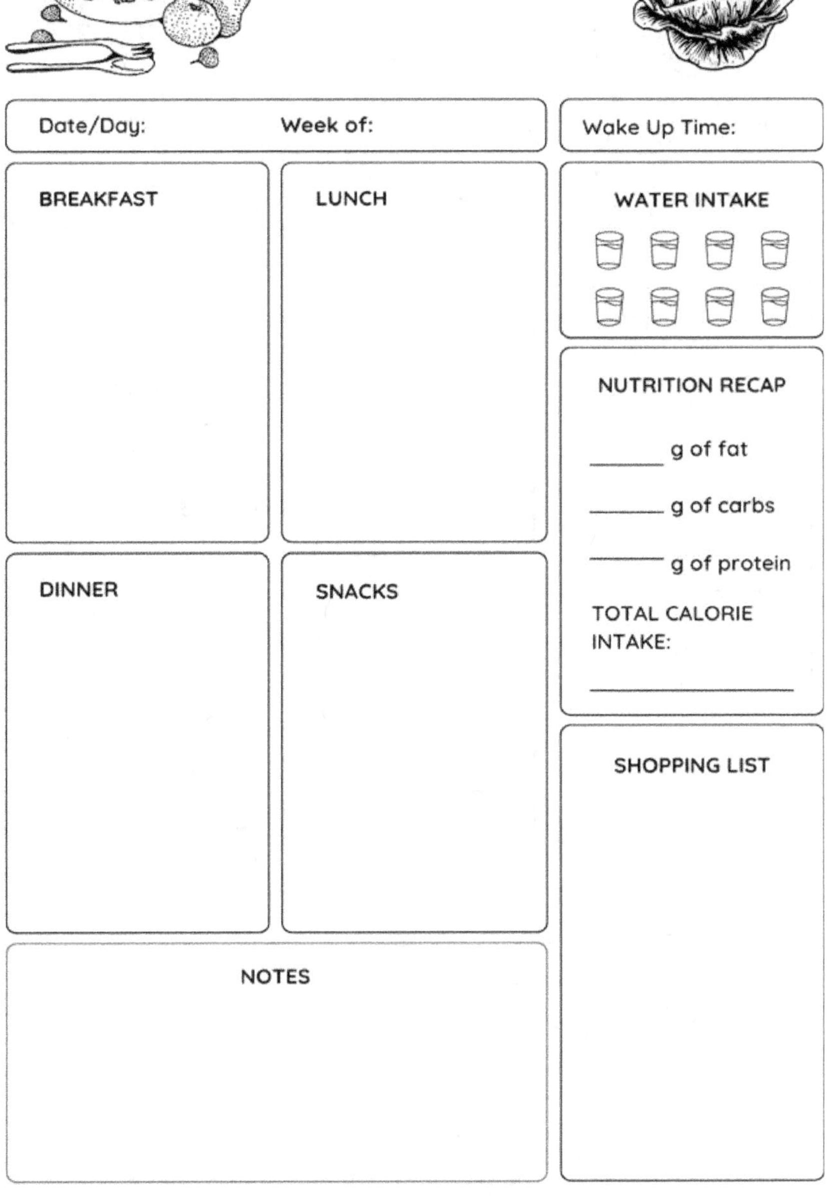

Date/Day: Week of:

Wake Up Time:

BREAKFAST

LUNCH

WATER INTAKE

NUTRITION RECAP

_______ g of fat

_______ g of carbs

_______ g of protein

TOTAL CALORIE INTAKE:

DINNER

SNACKS

SHOPPING LIST

NOTES

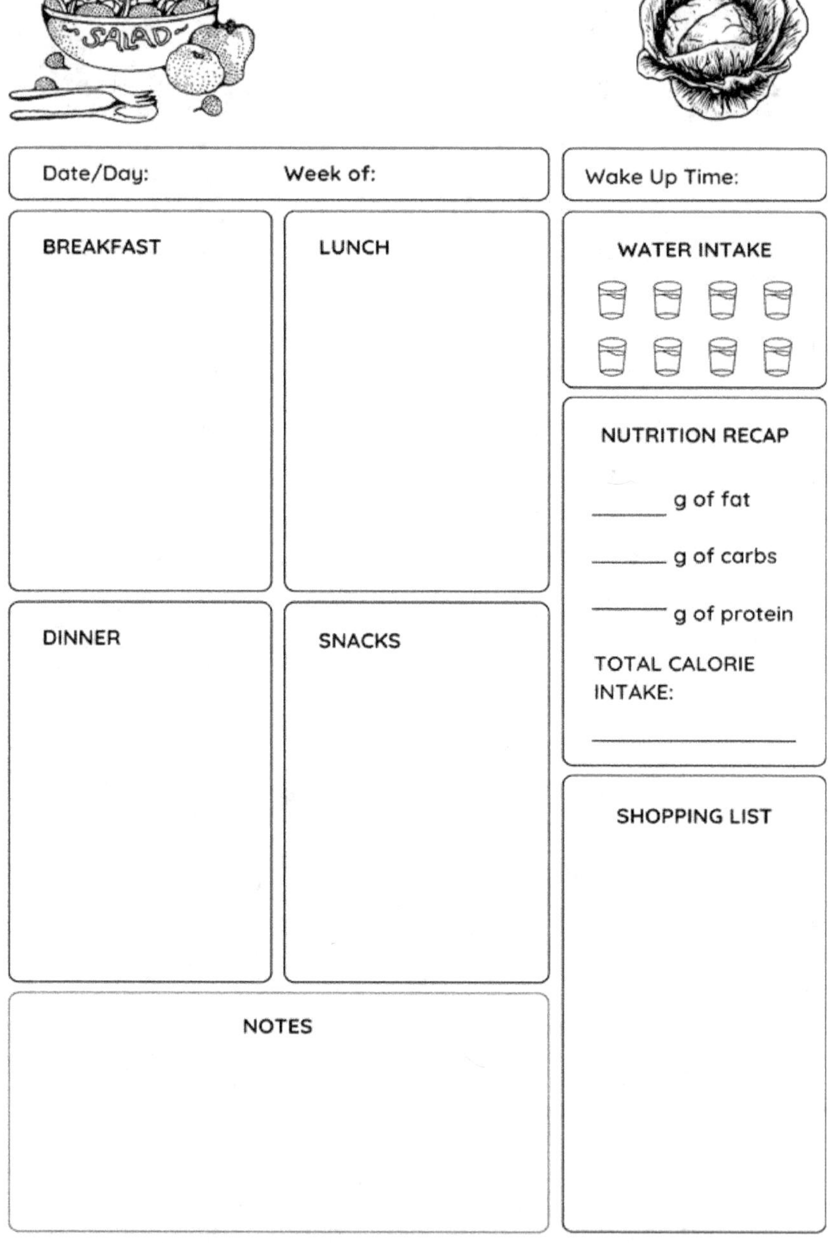

Date/Day:
Week of:
Wake Up Time:

BREAKFAST

LUNCH

WATER INTAKE

NUTRITION RECAP

________ g of fat

________ g of carbs

________ g of protein

TOTAL CALORIE
INTAKE:

____

DINNER

SNACKS

SHOPPING LIST

NOTES

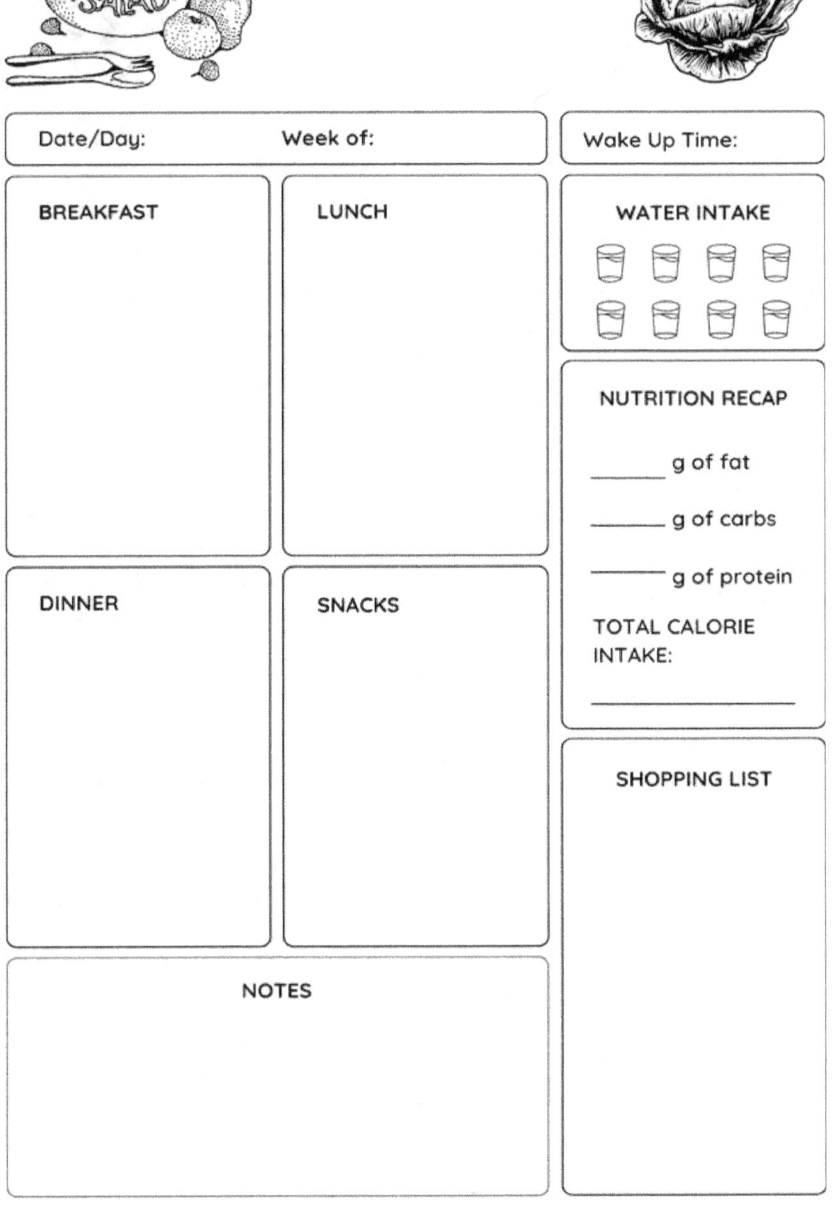

Date/Day:
Week of:
Wake Up Time:
BREAKFAST
LUNCH
WATER INTAKE
NUTRITION RECAP
_______ g of fat
_______ g of carbs
_______ g of protein
TOTAL CALORIE INTAKE:
DINNER
SNACKS
SHOPPING LIST
NOTES

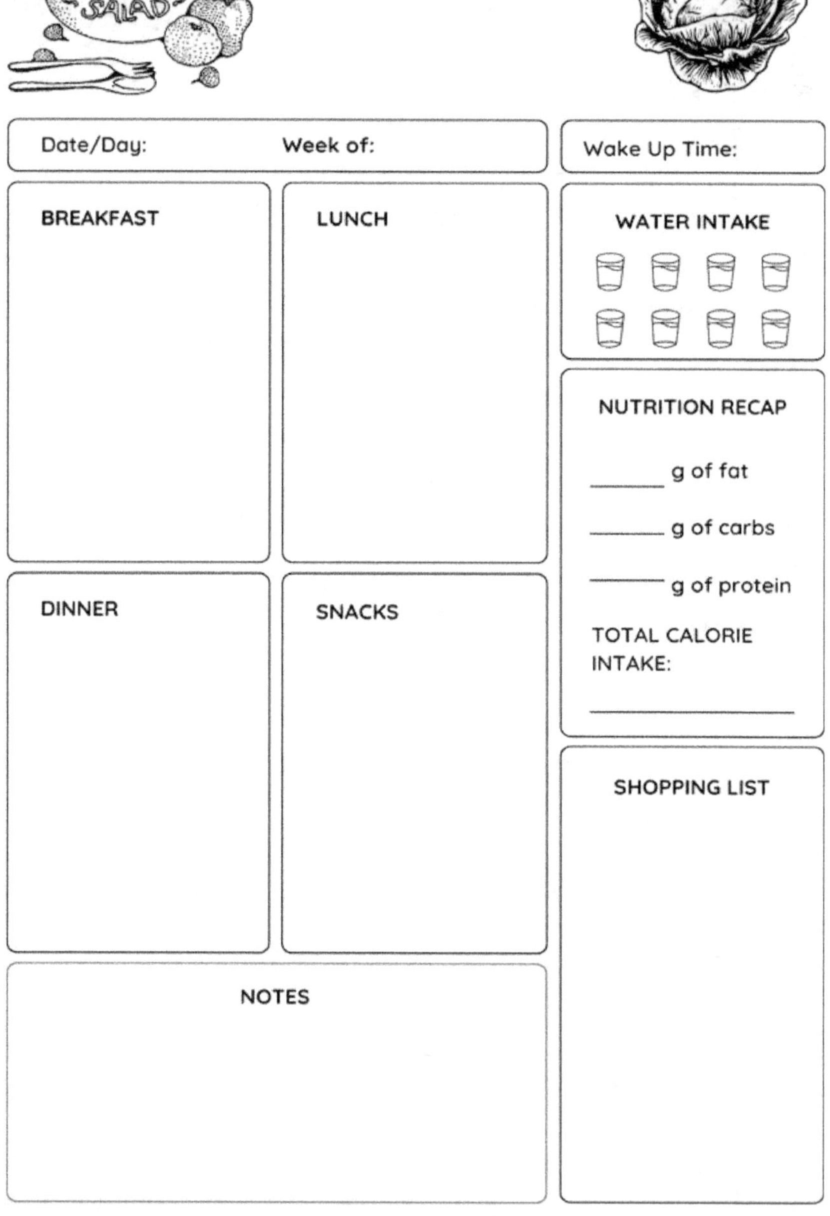

Date/Day: Week of:
BREAKFAST
LUNCH
DINNER
SNACKS
NOTES
Wake Up Time:
WATER INTAKE
NUTRITION RECAP
_______ g of fat
_______ g of carbs
_______ g of protein
TOTAL CALORIE INTAKE:
SHOPPING LIST

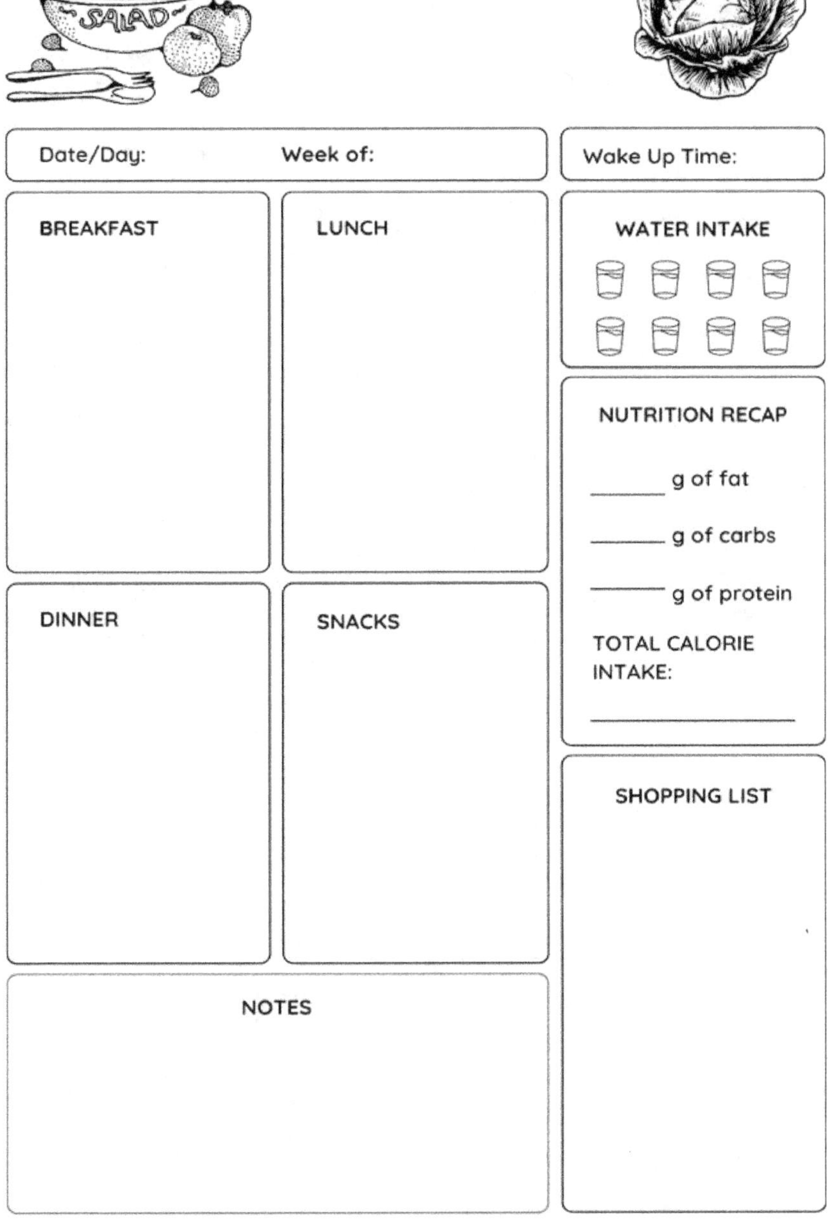

Date/Day: Week of:

Wake Up Time:

BREAKFAST

LUNCH

WATER INTAKE

NUTRITION RECAP

_______ g of fat

_______ g of carbs

_______ g of protein

TOTAL CALORIE INTAKE:

DINNER

SNACKS

SHOPPING LIST

NOTES

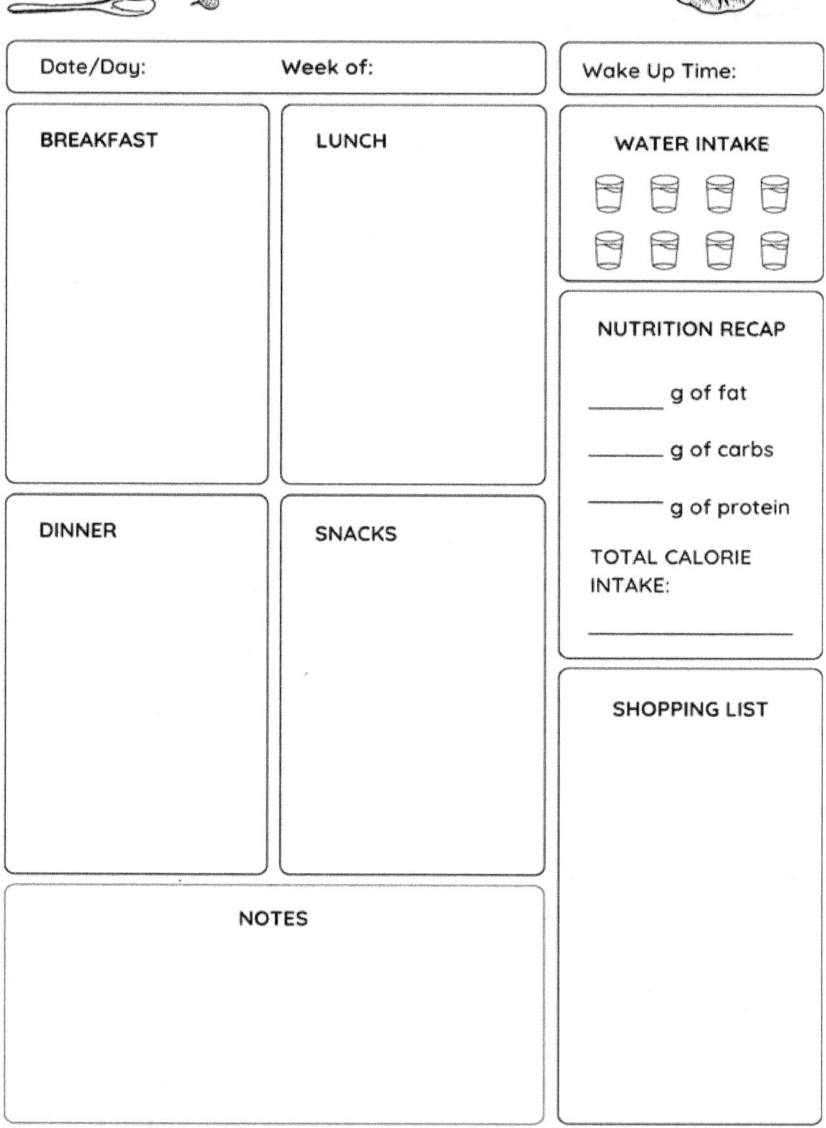

| Date/Day: | Week of: | Wake Up Time: |

BREAKFAST

LUNCH

WATER INTAKE

NUTRITION RECAP

________ g of fat

________ g of carbs

________ g of protein

TOTAL CALORIE INTAKE:

____

DINNER

SNACKS

SHOPPING LIST

NOTES

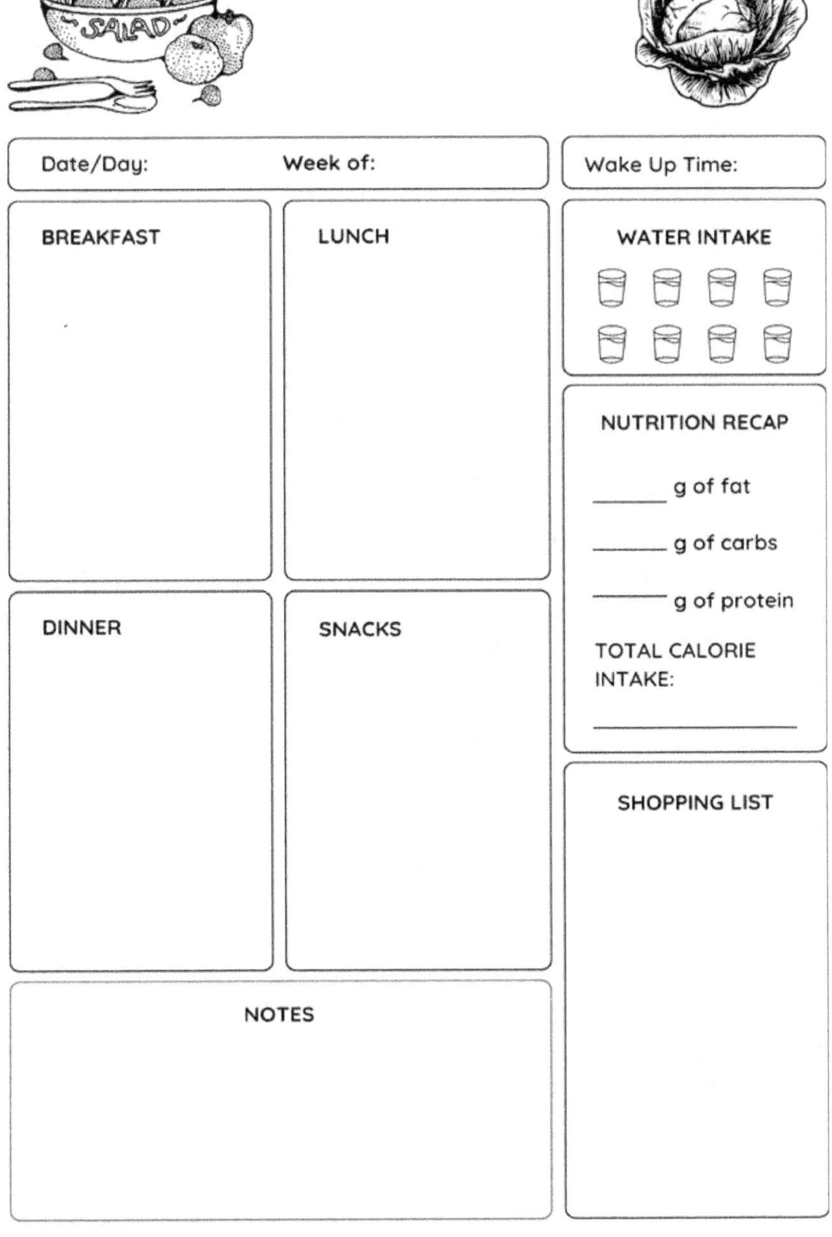

SALAD
Date/Day:
Week of:
Wake Up Time:
BREAKFAST
LUNCH
WATER INTAKE
NUTRITION RECAP
_______ g of fat
_______ g of carbs
_______ g of protein
TOTAL CALORIE INTAKE:
DINNER
SNACKS
SHOPPING LIST
NOTES